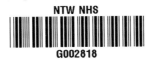

Speech and Language
Clinical Process and Practice

Second edition

Speech and Language Clinical Process and Practice

Second edition

Monica Bray
Speech and Language Therapy Group,
Leeds Metropolitan University

Alison Ross
Speech and Language Therapy Group,
Leeds Metropolitan University

Celia Todd
Speech and Language Therapist,
Cornwall Partnership Trust

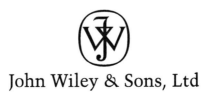

John Wiley & Sons, Ltd

Other Wiley Editorial Offices

John Wiley & Sons Inc., 111 River Street, Hoboken, NJ 07030, USA

Jossey-Bass, 989 Market Street, San Francisco, CA 94103-1741, USA

Wiley-VCH Verlag GmbH, Boschstr. 12, D-69469 Weinheim, Germany

John Wiley & Sons Australia Ltd, 42 McDougall Street, Milton, Queensland 4064, Australia

John Wiley & Sons (Asia) Pte Ltd, 2 Clementi Loop #02-01, Jin Xing Distripark, Singapore
129809

John Wiley & Sons Canada Ltd, 22 Worcester Road, Etobicoke, Ontario, Canada M9W 1L1

Wiley also publishes its books in a variety of electronic formats. Some content that appears in
print may not be available in electronic books.

A catalogue record for this book is available from the British Library

ISBN -13   978-1-861-56496-2 (pbk)

Contents

Preface to first edition

This book grew out of our own professional development as speech and language clinicians and our work with speech and language therapy students. Our experiences with students in clinical settings, workshops, seminars, tutorials and lectures have led us to an understanding of the struggles encountered and the questions asked by individuals who are in the transitional stage from student to qualified clinician. The only way to be ready to face the demands of professional practice and life-long learning is to thoroughly understand what the process and practice of clinical work actually are.

So the book is primarily for students, whom we have addressed throughout the text and considered when attempting to highlight the experiences and feelings they may encounter. But we also hope that it will be of value to others who work with students, and that some aspects of the book may be appreciated by experienced clinicians as an opportunity to revisit what is involved in therapy and professional practice. From feedback received when we have discussed the book with others, we suggest that it may provide a source of information for those just starting in the profession or returning to it after a time away. It is not intended to teach clinical skills or core knowledge, but to provide a combination of information, ideas, case iluustrations and concepts that we hope will guide students' professional practice. The ideas presented draw on the authors' vast range of reading, experience and thinking over many years, and represent our approaches and beliefs. It would be surprising if all clinicians agreed with everything we say, and where disagreement arises, this should provide the focus for healthy debate.

As the text does not attempt to provide a background of knowledge about speech pathology and therapy, linguistics, medical sciences, audiology, education, psychology or any of the many fields of theory that are important to the speech and language clinician, students are advised to use this book in tandem with their other learning experiences. We have concentrated on the areas that apply all of this learning and help to link theory and therapy – the clinical process and professional practice.

Clinical process is about the methods and actions used to effect positive change in people's communication functioning. Students commonly yearn to be told what to do when faced with a clinical problem. While demonstrating and explaining techniques such as ways of administering assessments, ways of interacting, and ways of shaping and reinforcing behaviours is essential, the appropriate and successful use of such methods must depend on a wealth of awareness, knowledge, attitudes and behaviours. It is these that we have tried to capture in this book.

Professional practice is about the context of our work, the people with whom we work, and the standards, attitudes and behaviours we adopt as clinicians in order to provide a high quality of care for people with communication disorders. This book endeavours to review the scope of speech and language practice.

The first two chapters set the scene by discussing the person of the speech and language clinician and the nature of intervention in general. Chapters 3 and 4 give the reader a chance to consider in depth the actual processes and practices that take place when clinician and client come together. Chapters 5 and 6 take a broader perspective, encouraging reflection on the role of the speech and language clinician in more detail. The place of and need for paperwork to support clinical practice is discussed in Chapter 7, and finally, in Chapter 8, we look at the transition from student to qualified clinician and the nature of continuing professional development. We would encourage students to read the book from cover to cover, but each chapter also stands alone, allowing readers to make choices about where they wish to focus. The many case discussions found through the book are based not on actual individuals but on an amalgamation of clients we have known through our many years of clinical practice.

While we acknowledge that speech and language clinicians may be male or female, we found that our initial attempts to signal this by he/she, his/her inhibited the flow for the reader, and therefore where gender has to be indicated, the female form has been chosen.

In learning we move from stage to stage, building on what we know, and moving from vague and uncertain formulations to clearer and more precise awareness. Readers will come to this book from different starting points, bringing with them their personal knowledge and experience. We hope it will enable them to move forward to a greater understanding of what goes on in clinical work.

Teaching and learning are two sides of the same coin. As we teach students, so we learn from them, thus expanding and increasing our own knowledge, skills and attitudes. This book is therefore dedicated to all our students, past, present and future, from whom we have learned so much and through whom we hope to continue to develop.

Monica Bray
Alison Ross
Celia Todd
April 1998

Preface to the second edition

It is 5 years since the publication of the first edition of this book and in that time much has changed in the professional practice of the speech and language clinician. The modernization of the National Health Service, the development of many initiatives by the government to alleviate disadvantage, and the changes in education led by the Department for Education and Skills have had a major impact on the work and roles undertaken by speech and language therapists. The registration of the profession under the auspices of the Health Professions Council and the growing demand for effective and evidence-based practice have led to a tightening of the specifications of what makes a speech and language professional and what constitutes good practice. This new edition has attempted to capture the current work practices and demands, and changes in Chapters 5, 6, 7 and 8 particularly reflect what is happening in the here and now.

When we first conceived of and wrote this book, it stood on its own in its attempts to capture the overall philosophies, ideas and concepts involved in clinical practice. It has since been joined by a number of other publications that have dealt with similar issues, often in more depth in particular areas or with a slightly different slant to ideas. We have drawn on the knowledge and expertise of the authors of these books and articles and refer to them liberally, and with thanks, in the current book, particularly in Chapters 1 and 2.

Despite the movement within the profession towards more consultative and collaborative work, we still believe that the student speech and language therapist needs a sound grasp of the basics of assessment and therapy in relation to the needs of specific clients with specific speech and language difficulties. Chapters 3 and 4 have remained, therefore, essentially the same, except for some updating and changes in the examples offered.

We hope that this second edition will enable student speech and language therapists and speech and language clinicians new to the field or returning to practice to keep up with what is happening in the field at this time. We would also like this book to be useful to speech and language clinical educators working to develop in their students the knowledge, skills and attitudes essential for today's professional person. It is the clinical educators who have been so forthcoming with ideas and suggestions in relation to clinical training that have helped the emergence of this second edition, and we thank them all for their valuable thoughts.

Alison Ross contributed to the planning of this new edition. Unfortunately due to other commitments she had to withdraw from writing the revisions. With her consent the parts she wrote in the first edition have been updated but much of her work remains unchanged.

Monica Bray
Celia Todd
May 2005

Chapter 1
The speech and language clinician

Before unravelling the mysteries of the processes, procedures, relationships and activities involved in managing communication disorders, it is helpful to take some time to consider the characteristics and roles of the professionals who are central to this field. These are the people who, in this book, we have chosen to call speech and language clinicians. To build up a picture of these people we will try to answer a few questions about their work:

- What is the focus and range of their work?
- What are the roles they play?
- Where do they work?
- Whom do they help?
- What approaches are applied in their work?
- What knowledge, skills and attitudes are special to their work?

The following is intended only as an introduction to the more comprehensive discussion that follows later in the book.

Focus and range of the work of the speech and language clinician

'Logopaedist', 'speech–language pathologist', 'speech pathologist', 'speech–language pathologist and audiologist', 'speech and language therapist', 'orthophonist', 'phonoaudiologist', 'speech therapist', 'speech clinician' and 'communication clinician' are some of the titles, or the English translations of titles, that are used by various nations (American Speech-Language-Hearing Association [ASHA] and International Association of Logopedics and Phoniatrics [IALP] 1994) to denote a professional who is specifically qualified to work with individuals or groups of people who have speech and language disorders. In reality, the work will not be restricted to a narrow focus on speech and language, but will encompass wider aspects of human communication as well as the functions and processes that are related to speech and language, such as swallowing and hearing.

Cultural, political, financial, education and training, employment and other national differences mean that the emphasis of the work practice of speech and language clinicians varies from country to country. In some countries, speech and language clinicians concentrate on children with speech and language disorders, including those disorders that are secondary to deafness and special education; in others the work is hospital-based and concerns disorders associated with medical conditions. In some countries the work involves both child and adult disorders in schools, hospitals and other settings. Sometimes the speech and language clinician will be qualified in another field as well, such as audiology and hearing therapy, special education or another rehabilitation specialism, such as physiotherapy, occupational therapy or ophthalmology (Lesser 1992). The methods that speech and language clinicians use, including the degree of formality in their methods, will also differ. There is, however, a great deal of common ground between speech and language clinicians in their commitment to the prevention, assessment, intervention, management and scientific study of communication and associated disorders. Although this book is likely to have a British bias, we endeavour to refer to a range of practices that are familiar to, or can be readily applied in, other nations.

The way in which speech and language clinicians work is evolving and is likely to continue to change with changing social concepts, values and government-led initiatives. A variety of roles and working practices has emerged and been added to the 'traditional' role of therapist so that the clinician may, within a working week, undertake many of the roles in Figure 1.1.

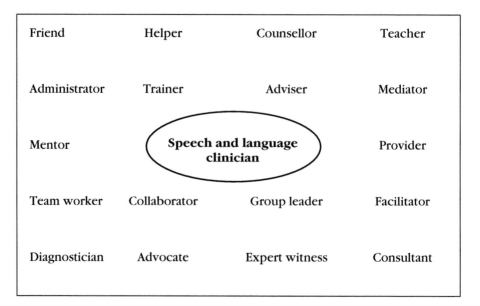

Friend	Helper	Counsellor	Teacher
Administrator	Trainer	Adviser	Mediator
Mentor	Speech and language clinician		Provider
Team worker	Collaborator	Group leader	Facilitator
Diagnostician	Advocate	Expert witness	Consultant

Figure 1.1 The roles of the speech and language clinician.

For example, on a Monday morning, the clinician may be in a school *collaborating* with the class teacher and drawing up a joint plan to enable a child to access the curriculum more easily. She may spend time modelling techniques and *training* the learning support assistant. In the afternoon she may be the *group leader* in a social skills group for children from the school, and at the end of the day she may be part of a *team* meeting in which one particular child is discussed. On Tuesday this same clinician may work *as part of a team* with young adults with learning difficulty, where she may act as the *friend and advocate* for a particular young man who is trying to get an appointment to see a careers adviser. She may be *providing* a communication book to *support* the interaction between this young man and the careers adviser. Later, she may *facilitate* a group meeting within the college that this young man attends in order to help others with learning difficulties to talk about their hopes for the future. On Wednesday she may visit the home of one of the children she has seen at the local community clinic. Here she will listen to and reflect and summarize the worries of the parents of a young child who stammers, thus acting as a *counsellor*, enabling them to express their concerns. Later she may watch a video they have made of themselves interacting with their child and will help them consider how they may reduce some of the pressure to speak for their child. She will *advise* them on ways of talking and reinforcing their child's speaking in order to reduce the stammering, thus *empowering* them to be their child's main 'therapists'.

In the afternoon a colleague who is new to working with children who stammer may *consult* her about the process and she will act as a *mentor* to this colleague to help develop the specialist skills needed in this area. On Thursday, the clinician may spend the day in the community clinic where much of her time will be given to *teaching* skills to children who have speech or language difficulties and again modelling these to the parents. Throughout the week, case notes will be written up, phone calls made, discussion undertaken and at the end of the week reports will need to be written, plans made and materials adapted, and other *administration* will be undertaken. A clinician working predominantly with adults with acquired difficulties (people with speech and language problems after stroke, accident or progressive disorder) would also be engaged in as wide a range of roles throughout the week as our imaginary individual above.

Speech and language clinical contexts

'Clinician' is the most universally appropriate term to describe the manner of work of the specialist who provides care for people with speech and language and related problems. It is selected in preference to 'pathologist', which implies a study of disorder or disease without intervention, or 'therapist', which suggests a concentration on treatment. The term 'clinician' may conjure up images of work in medical settings, either at the hospital bedside or in health clinics, and a primary concern for presenting conditions and disorders. However, most importantly, it conveys the message that the specialist concerned is objective and applies a scientific, problem-solving approach to the observation, evaluation and management of people – the 'clients'.

As the medical model of service delivery has shifted to a social model of practice (see later), so the speech and language clinician has come out of the hospital or clinic into the wider community. This does not mean that the more 'traditional' settings are not still the focus of much of our work, but more and more we are following the client into his or her living or working space. So, as a speech and language clinician you may work in hospital wards and hospital or health centre clinics, but there are other places where you can contact clients. You might make contact at their place of residence, perhaps the family home or a care home, or in the place they go to in the daytime, such as a day centre or school. You may also work in other settings, including resource centres that provide a service for augmentative communication system users. To help answer the question 'Where do they work?', the Royal College of Speech and Language Therapists (RCSLT 1996) has compiled a list of settings or service locations, which is presented below. From this you should gain a sense of the breadth of the possible contexts of client-related work:

- acute hospital settings
- rehabilitation centres
- community clinics
- specialist outpatient centres
- day centres, including adult training centres, social education centres and resource centres
- supported living or group homes
- domiciliary (i.e. visits to the home of the client)
- day nurseries
- child development centres
- mainstream schools
- resourced schools
- special schools, including classes and units
- language units, including schools and classes
- nursery schools.
- further educational settings
- clinics within higher educational establishments.

There is a range of types of organization in which speech and language clinicians are employed, in both this and other countries. Among the many possible employment settings for speech and language clinicians are:

- public sector organizations, such as a National Health Service or a social or welfare service
- individual or group private practice

- voluntary sector organizations funded by grants and charities, e.g. for people with visual impairment or with hearing loss, for people who are brain-injured, or for children with a specific language impairment, and more.

Although working practices may vary according to the requirements of the employing organization, you will find that the values shared and practised by speech and language clinicians are fundamentally the same.

The speech and language client/service user

Speech and language clinicians are concerned with *individuals* and groups of individuals, and their abilities in communication and related areas such as swallowing and hearing. They also work with carers and involved others who are themselves concerned with these individuals or groups. The use of the term 'client' rather than 'patient' is chosen to avoid any implication that the person concerned is ill or has a medical condition, or that the treatment given should be merely symptom related. This means that there is an acknowledgement that problems such as the strained voice of a teacher or the delayed language development of a child may have little or no association with a medical condition, and further, that each of these cases may require intervention that goes beyond instruction related to the observed impairment, i.e. in vocal exercises for the teacher or in language production tasks for the child. The intervention is likely instead to be based on changing underlying influences such as the environment, listening skills or attitudes.

There is no intention to ignore the fact that many speech and language clients do have a communication problem resulting from a medical condition, such as Parkinson's disease, stroke, head injury, cerebral palsy, hearing loss, cleft palate or laryngectomy. These people will need the support of medical personnel. However, each of these people is far more than the outcome of a medical problem. They have different backgrounds, values and attitudes, experiences, physical characteristics and behaviours, and all these factors, as well as their medical condition, will contribute to the way in which the individual deals with his or her ability to communicate. This should be accounted for in the management decisions of medical and other personnel. The client should not be viewed merely as part of a medical problem, and should not be treated just like the last person who presented with the same diagnosis.

The choice of the term 'client' rather than patient also places the individual with the communication problem in an active rather than a passive role in the relationship with the clinician and the speech and language service provided. In the world of business, 'client' is often used interchangeably with 'customer', 'consumer' and 'user' (Harrow and Shaw 1992). *Service user* reflects the wider role of the speech and language clinician in the education and training of involved others. As a consumer of the service, the client is becoming increasingly well informed and is more involved in decision-making about his or her own health-care needs. The client has choices to indicate his or her preferences and to take or leave the care that is offered (Kineen 1994). These concepts similarly underpin care provision, including speech and language services. The clinician will establish mutually agreed contracts with her clients, in which all clients have equal rights to be provided with the best possible quality of care and to be involved in management decisions. This is considered further in the discussion of the client-centred approach, below.

Speech and language disorder classification

While never losing sight of the individuality of each client, for convenience, speech and language clinicians tend to classify communication disorders according to the presenting problem. This involves broad categories, such as *developmental*, indicating that the problem has been present in some way since infancy, *acquired*, indicating that the onset of the problem was after infancy, or *progressive*, indicating a deterioration associated with either a developmental or an acquired condition. There have been several attempts to categorize the many and varied types of communication and related disorders that can occur. Two classification systems are given below.

Classification of presenting disorders (RCSLT 1996)

- Acquired language disorder/adult aphasia
- Acquired childhood aphasia
- Developmental speech and language disorders
- Written language disorders
  - developmental
  - acquired
- Developmental dysarthria
- Acquired dysarthria
- Acquired phonetic disorders
- Dysphonia
- Dysfluency
- Dysphagia
- Eating and drinking difficulties in children.

Classification of linguistic pathologies (Crystal and Varley 1998)

- Cognitive disorders, e.g. thought disorders, autism and learning difficulties
- Language disorders, e.g. aphasia, and developmental language disorder
- Apraxia
- Dysarthria
- Disorders of voice, e.g. vocal misuse and laryngectomy
- Disorders of fluency, e.g. cluttering and stuttering

- Disorders of articulation, e.g. cleft palate and glossectomy
- Hearing impairment
- Agnosia.

Approaches applied in speech and language clinical practice

Earlier, when we looked at the roles that you might play, we touched on some of the approaches that would be used within these roles. The important thing to remember is that speech and language clinicians do not adopt a narrow, symptom-based approach to practice. Instead it is agreed that a *holistic* approach is essential in the assessment and intervention of communication problems. Not only should the clinician endeavour to address any voice, fluency, speech and language, or swallowing problem that presents, but she must also consider the wider effects and implications of the problem. However, other influences are at work when decisions are being made about approaches within practice. Issues such as the current philosophy of client-centredness and social models of health care, government edicts linked to quality assurance and clinical governance, professional values and ethics, and regulatory body demands all drive and mould decisions.

Communication and related disorders can lead to a loss of independence, a change in lifestyle, confusion, frustration, failure at school, adverse reactions from others and difficulty with relationships. As the disorder will normally be greater than the sum of the presenting features, the clinician needs to look at every contributing factor and determine the wide-ranging intervention that could help to alleviate the disorder. Management decisions should be based on a wealth of knowledge about the person, the problem complex, the communication experience and needs of the individual and, not least, his or her wishes for change. The following examples illustrate how decision-making is based on more than the overt features or the disorder classification:

1. An adult with a decline in written language skills after a stroke, who had never previously achieved or needed high-level literacy skills, would not be expected to contemplate more than the simplest reading and writing task.
2. A person who stammers and is comfortable with his or her image of self and dysfluent speech would not be a candidate for therapy.
3. A child with a language delay who is teased at school or whose parents are overanxious and inappropriately correcting disordered speech attempts might be given higher priority than a child who does not have to cope with the added problems.

A client-centred approach to therapy, first put forward by Rogers in the 1940s (Rogers 1951), is advocated by most speech and language clinicians and is promoted in this book. This does not mean that more directed approaches are not considered. Unlike directive approaches, where the role of the clinician or therapist applies rather prescribed methods to achieve change, the client-centred approach emphasizes the role of the therapist as a *facilitator*. The therapist, in this case the speech and language clinician, encourages clients to:

- explore aspects of themselves and ways of relating to others
- practise new behaviours
- change their perceptions, attitudes and performance
- engage with the clinician in joint problem-solving around their difficulties
- take responsibility for their own therapy programme.

Throughout this process of development, reformulation and change, the speech and language clinician works in partnership with the client. As a speech and language clinician, you will draw on professional knowledge and skills to guide the collection of evidence, and to inform, clarify and provide the opportunity for the client to practise different behaviours. In addition, you will offer a context of trust and empathy within which the client is *empowered*. This means that the client adopts a sense of ownership of the therapy process and shares the responsibility for the outcomes. Thus, we have an approach in which clinical decisions are a joint venture between the client and the clinician. The approach stresses the importance of negotiation and choice, including choice about whether or not to receive treatment and choice about the direction of treatment.

Of particular importance in helping the client to effect change is the role of the clinician in listening, demystifying and clarifying. This involves attending to the person's view of him- or herself, taking account of all the factors contributing to the disorder, and explaining and helping him or her to appreciate the nature of the problems, the alternative ways of addressing them, and the prognosis or outcomes to expect from the choices made.

Implicit in this therapy approach, and a general underpinning principle of speech and language clinicians, is that the intended outcomes of therapy constitute positive change not 'cure'. As Finkelstein (1993) reminds us, the concept of cure is determined by standards and beliefs about what is normal. Speech and language clinicians do not seek to cure. They aim to offer optimal help in changing behaviours and attitudes within the boundaries appropriate for the individual, and to enable clients to attain the best quality of life that they can within their own normality. This may be particularly difficult to come to terms with for some clients. A man who has an acquired disability, such as dysarthria after a head injury, may have a previous construct of self that he aspires to rebuild. A mother may expect her child who has learning difficulties to achieve the same level of language functioning as children of the same age who do not have learning difficulties. These situations will require a sensitive response and carefully managed support from the clinician.

It is not too difficult to appreciate how the client-centred approach works for adults who possess a reasonable level of cognitive skills and can comprehend and express ideas, consider alternatives, analyse and problem solve. But what happens in the case of a person who has severe linguistic impairment, learning difficulties or cognitive deficit, or who is an infant? In these cases a parent, relative, friend or, where none of these is available, a professional or other person might be called upon to act as a proxy or advocate for the client. As Brechin and Swain (1988) explain, advocacy is based on the principle of creating opportunities for self-determination, i.e. the power to make a decision for oneself. Within formal structures or informally, the advocate has responsibility for promoting decisions that will enable the client to have greater autonomy. Decisions should not be based on what might be easiest for, or preferred by, a carer, service or other agency. In this way, the advocate who contributes to speech and language management decisions should be the voice of the client.

Professional judgement

In addition to the role of the client in determining the change that should be brought about, there are other essential ingredients in the decision-making process that must be noted. These are the competencies required of a speech and language therapist as laid down by the professional and regulatory bodies, the professional judgement of the speech and language clinician, and the availability of provision and resources (Leahy 1989).

Speech and language therapy competencies

The way in which speech and language clinicians practise in the UK is defined and guided by sets of principles laid down by both the professional body (RCSLT) and the registering body (Health Professions' Council – HPC). These bodies have as their aims both the development of the profession and professionals and the safety and well-being of the clients. To ensure these, a set of principles is laid down, a few of which are itemized below.

The RCSLT suggests that the following attributes are vital to working as a speech and language therapist (RCSLT 2003c):

- a desire to improve clients' quality of life
- a commitment to the empowerment of others
- a sensitivity to other cultures and religions.

The Health Professions Council (HPC 2003) considers it important that speech and language clinicians:

- know the professional and personal scope of their practice and are able to make referrals

- are able to work in partnership with other professionals
- are able to demonstrate effective appropriate skills in communicating.

The professional judgement of the speech and language clinician

Although the preferences of the individual client have a high priority, decisions must be made in the light of what is realistic and possible in terms of theoretical and clinical knowledge. Speech and language theory and practice are an ever-growing body of understanding, supported by research and evidence of efficacy for particular intervention strategies and it is the duty, as defined by both the RCSLT and the HPC, of the speech and language clinician to base management decisions on strong evidence of the efficacy of strategies used and to ensure as far as possible that the therapy programme is viable and well researched (Reilly 2004). At the same time, the experience of each clinician will bring boundless evidence of practice that is appropriate and of value to clients.

The availability of provision and resources

Every service will have limits to its resources. This will affect how much time you can spend with clients, when you can spend the time and the type of intervention you can offer. You can only offer what is possible within the resources available and in your power to provide, but also, whatever you offer must be given in fairness to other service users. You cannot merely respond to demand and, while listening to and remaining in touch with the client, it is important not to over-promise (Kineen 1994).

Public promotion

As Byers Brown and Gilbert (1989) remind us, communication handicap is a product of the whole community, not only of the individual who has the disorder. A person with a communication problem is part of a social context within which both the individual and the community react and adapt in a variety of ways. To reduce the occurrence and effects of handicap, people who are likely to interact with individuals with potential and actual handicap need to be targeted. To this end another aspect of the work of speech and language clinicians is that of promoting public understanding of communication problems and people who have communication problems. In addition to responding to general opportunities to increase the knowledge and under-standing of the population at large, clinicians might focus on selected groups who have contact with people with communication disorder by, for example:

- providing a series of talks and leading discussions with sets of children in their schools
- running workshops for staff of care homes for elderly people.

In these cases the client is not a specific person but a population group that is affected or at risk of being affected by communication disorder.

The aim of the speech and language clinician is to provide 'the best possible care for those who suffer from communication handicap' (Byers Brown and Gilbert 1989). To achieve this diagnostic assessment, remedy, support, information and guidance have to be made available for the benefit of both those who 'suffer' and those who care for them. The key words explaining this management process are *assessment*, *treatment* and *advice* or *information*. These are not separate entities, as later chapters explain, but interdependent aspects of the clinical process.

Constant *hypothesis testing*, i.e. making and verifying tentative propositions, is central to the assessment, treatment, and advice and information-giving involved in clinical management, e.g.:

- You might observe that a child is uncommunicative in the clinic and so put forward a hypothesis that he or she is uncommunicative in other situations. You can then test this hypothesis by asking the mother or teacher about communication in the home and school, or by observing the child outside the clinic setting.
- You might form a hypothesis that a young child's language skills would improve if therapy concentrated on working with the mother. You can then introduce a programme involving the mother and later assess whether change has occurred.
- You might hypothesize that an adult's language deficit is exacerbated by a hearing loss. After referral for audiometric assessment and subsequent fitting of a hearing aid you can monitor any improvement in language to test your hypothesis.

In this way, you explore the communication problem and the needs of the individual, assess whether intervention is required and what intervention would be most appropriate, and then evaluate the degree to which the range of aspects of your intervention has achieved what you and the client intended.

Knowledge, skills and attitudes of speech and language clinicians

All health professionals are obliged to deal effectively with a growing body of scientific, technical and professional knowledge and to be concerned with the well-being of the whole person, which entails (Higgs and Titchen 2000):

- understanding complex human desires for dignity, independence and support
- appreciating concerns, needs, frames of reference of clients
- the ability to cope with pain and frailty
- the ability to deal with ethical dilemmas.

So what does the speech and language clinician do that is special? As a speech and language clinician, you will not be the only professional involved with people with disorders of communication or swallowing difficulties. A schoolteacher helps children with reading, writing or spoken language problems. A dietitian advises people on food consistencies and quantities. A psychologist offers support to the parents of children with autism. A doctor recommends ways of overcoming a voice disorder. A nurse helps with the feeding problems arising from neurological disorder. A volunteer visitor offers a person, who is language-impaired after a stroke support and practice in speech, comprehension, reading and writing. A care assistant encourages the communication skills of elderly people in a care home. However, it is the speech and language clinician who is enabled through a range of specific learning and professional and practical development to bring together a particular set of knowledge, attitudes and skills that is different from those of the other professions mentioned. You will be dependent on the different specialist sets of knowledge and skills of these experts. You will work with these others (see Chapter 5) to optimize the change in communication that you hope your clients will achieve.

There are four main disciplines at the core of our learning as speech and language clinicians: psychology, medical sciences, linguistics, and speech and language pathology. In addition, you will draw on learning from many other fields, including education and sociology. The knowledge, skills and attitudes required by speech and language clinicians are accumulated through reading, listening and discussion, and through observation and practice. The learning of speech and language clinicians encompasses, for example:

- human behaviour and how people perceive, learn and make decisions
- language, language use and language development
- interpersonal skills, attitudes and reactions
- development from embryo to old age
- multicultural society and the policies that govern society
- anatomy and physiology, and medical conditions
- disorders of communication and their management.

The skills that we need to acquire are equally far ranging, e.g. planning, negotiating, assessing, explaining, observing, decision-making, teaching, counselling and record keeping. The clinician also needs to develop and refine attitudes, including enthusiasm, adaptability, empathy, reliability and willingness to promote the needs of clients. This does not mean that other professionals and non-professionals do not apply some of the knowledge, skills and attitudes that are applied by speech and language professionals, but they will apply them to a greater or lesser extent and in a different combination. It is important to recognize that certain abilities or attributes are common to other personnel as well as speech and language clinicians, but these personnel have different roles and responsibilities and need their own special combination of what are often called competencies.

Not only do speech and language clinicians develop a core of skills, attitudes and knowledge that can be transferred to new contexts, but also as they concentrate on a special field further knowledge and skills specific to the area are accumulated. Davies and van der Gaag (Davies and van der Gaag 1992, van der Gaag and Davies 1992a, 1992b), in their studies of three groups of clinicians (one working with children, one with child and adult learning difficulties, and one with elderly people/acquired neurological disorders), show that some knowledge, attitudes and skills are common to all speech and language clinicians, and some are more specific to a particular group of specialist speech and language clinicians. In both pre- and post-qualification professional development, you will acquire knowledge, attitudes and skills that are specific to specialist areas of work, e.g. voice, hearing impairment, learning disability, head injury or augmentative communication, as well as knowledge, attitudes and skills that are common to more than one area of work.

It is not easy to define the make-up of a speech and language clinician. In a discussion emphasizing the importance of viewing the client/customer as an individual and the ways to ensure that their needs are best met by the clinician, Kineen (1994), referring to the work of Parasuraman et al. (1985), suggests a range of attributes that should be promoted. These are equally relevant to the relationship between speech and language clinicians and their clients and are defined below to stimulate an awareness of the many facets of the speech and language clinician and the quality of service that should be provided:

1. **Responsiveness**: a promptness and willingness to support.
2. **Competence**: having the required skills and knowledge.
3. **Access**: providing availability and ease of contact.
4. **Communication**: keeping the client informed in a way that they understand, and listening.
5. **Courtesy**: politeness, respect, consideration and friendliness.
6. **Security**: confidential in manner and in recording and reporting.
7. **Credibility**: trustworthiness, honesty and keeping the best interest of the client at heart.
8. **Understanding and knowing**: understanding the client's needs, constantly reviewing one's own skills and attitudes, and actively evaluating intervention.
9. **Tangibility**: ensuring appropriate physical aspects of facilities and materials.

A primary aim of this book is to support the developing professional in the rather daunting task of acquiring the attitudes, knowledge and skills that contribute to being an effective speech and language clinician.

Chapter 2
Intervention

Intervention is a decisive act to bring about change. It can be seen as either positive or negative and occurs both in a professional context and as part of everyday life. Examples of intervention are:

- seeking or giving advice
- stopping or starting an argument
- dieting or overeating to change body shape
- enabling a friend to express feelings of grief after suffering loss or injury
- introducing new rules into the household in order to keep rooms tidy.

Bunning (2004) sees intervention as a cycle as shown in Figure 2.1, which should be based on sound professional or clinical judgements and must be driven by a rationale or hypothesis. The clinician must be knowledgeable and have good problem-solving skills in order to use the assessment process to make decisions about therapy. The evaluation aspect of the cycle demands a clinician who is reflective and self-aware.

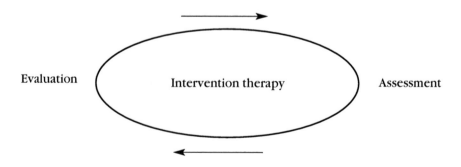

Figure 2.1 Cycle of intervention. (After Bunning 2004.)

The decision to take a particular course of action must be justified in terms of an underlying theory and knowledge of practice and the potential appropriateness of the action for the specific client. Thus, there are ethical values that must be taken into account. You would neither decide against treatment nor introduce a particular type of treatment if you perceived that the outcome would be harmful or ineffective. When the speech and language clinician intervenes, it is with a view to effecting positive change, whether in the communication behaviour or attitude of the person him- or herself, in altering the way others relate to the person, or in finding out more about the person to inform subsequent intervention further.

The following examples illustrate something of the scope of speech and language intervention:

- Discussing the problems of a non-communicating child with his or her teacher and agreeing the most appropriate way to encourage his or her communication.
- Setting up a group to develop the communication skills of adults with learning disability within a social context.
- Supporting Partners of People with Aphasia in Relationships and Conversation (SPPARC) (Lock et al. 2001) to help people who have aphasia and their partners to communicate better.
- Metaphon (Dean and Howell 1986, Dean et al. 1995) to enable children with phonological delay to understand the nature of their speech output.
- Using a multifaceted approach to helping adults who stammer, such as that proposed by Turnbull and Stewart (1999).
- Early Birds, which is an early intervention package developed by the National Autistic Association for parents and professionals (www.nas.org.uk).
- Referring a child with a phonological disorder for an ear, nose and throat (ENT) opinion and audiological assessment, with the possibility of being fitted with and trained in the use of a hearing aid to improve speech reception and processing.
- Disseminating information packages to care assistants in nursing homes or running workshops to help them to promote an effective communication environment for the elderly people with whom they work.
- Providing counselling opportunities for a person to reflect on the factors contributing to his or her voice disorder.
- Joining with other professionals to set up a book club for parents of children who may be at risk of failing to develop language to the level of their peers.

Decision-making and intervention

How do you know what intervention is appropriate, what to do, and where and when to start? The answer lies in what Byng (1995) calls 'clinical intuition, or the outcome of experience'. This is not something that a clinician has been born with, but something that develops from a multitude of learning and problem-solving skills. Judgements made about the range of types of intervention to apply, their timing and ordering, and the ways in which you will use them in a particular situation will be based on your individual knowledge and experience of intervention at that time. You will be dependent on what you have read, learned, seen, discussed, adapted and tried in the past: 'Rome was not built in a day'. Even the most experienced clinician will have once lacked knowledge, practice experience and confidence, and will constantly add to, draw on, practise and appraise her current body of knowledge and skills to meet new situations. Professional development does not stop when you gain a qualification to practise, but carries on throughout your professional life. So, keep reading, watching, talking, practising and evaluating.

Speech and language clinicians constantly evaluate the effectiveness of therapy. Unfortunately, much of the reported evidence of effectiveness that is available is anecdotal rather than research based, and there is little agreement about what aspects of intervention are effective (see Enderby and Emerson 1995). However, it is essential that the speech and language clinician be conversant with the current literature in the area and know the status of the evidence around the usefulness of a particular approach (Reilly [2004] identifies four different levels of evidence: 1 = systematic review; 2 = randomized controlled study; 3 controlled trial without randomization; 4 = opinion of respected authority). Even so, two clinicians might differ in their opinion as to what should be done. For a particular child referred with a language disorder, one clinician might, with justifiable reasons, say that intervention should consist solely of parental discussion and guidance. A second clinician might, with equal theoretical argument, say that intervention should concentrate on involving the child in a controlled learning environment with the clinician.

Intervention will be guided by a number of principles. Although there is some personal decision-making in the choice of approach, it is no longer acceptable simply to follow your 'gut feeling' when deciding how to proceed. The principles that will guide you will derive from a number of areas of guidance.

Clinical guidelines

The Royal College of Speech and Language Therapists (RCSLT 2004a) has brought out a set of clinical guidelines to support clinicians in their decisions. These have been developed through consultation with experts in different fields of speech and language and swallowing difficulties, and also by written evidence in the areas. They are an attempt therefore to provide less experienced clinicians with the evidence needed to support their chosen approach. Some examples from the field of disorders of fluency are:

- Patterns of communication within a family influence a child's developing speech, language and fluency skills. Observation of the child interacting with significant others may be documented in order to ascertain whether changes in interaction would be beneficial to the child's fluency.
- Therapy approaches (for adults) include fluency shaping, stammer-more-fluently approaches, and psychological therapies and communication skills training. These are not mutually exclusive.

Speech and language therapy competencies

The aim of this project (RCSLT 2003c) has been to try to define what are essential knowledge, skills and values in the profession. These have now been consolidated into a set of core competencies as well as competencies required within each defined area of work, e.g. the following are some core competencies.

Core values, beliefs, attitudes

- Commitment to an involvement in continuous professional development
- Commitment to working as part of a team in support of the client
- Willingness to accept own professional limitations
- Core knowledge base.

Knowledge and skills related to specific client groups

- Adult-acquired communication disorders
- Adult dysfluency
- Adult learning difficulties
- Childhood communication disorders
- Cleft palate
- Deafness
- Disorders of feeding
- Voice disorders
- Mental health disorder (and so on)
- Knowledge of legal frameworks and local systems
- Core skills
- Critical thinking skills such as integration of data from different sources, synthesis of information, generating hypotheses
- Caseload/workload management such as prioritizing
- Computer literacy.

National Service Frameworks

The government has produced a number of frameworks based on the NHS values of modernization, breaking down of professional barriers and partnership between agencies (www.dh.gov.uk). The National Service Framework (NSF) for Older People (Department of Health or DoH 2001b), for example, has eight standards to which agencies must conform. These include:

- Reducing age discrimination
- Providing client-centred care
- In stroke care ensuring that people are referred to a specialist stroke team.

For more discussion on how government policy affects service delivery, see Hickman (2002).

Person-centred planning

Hickman (2002) discusses the shift in focus from the professional to the client. In a consumer-driven society, the client and his or her significant others are central to decision-making about any interventions. The professional has a role in being able to educate and give options to the client and his family but what, when and how intervention will occur will rest on joint agreement, not the professional's wishes.

Goals of intervention

Bunning (2004) identifies a number of general goals that will influence decision-making. These are adapted from the work of Byng et al. (2000) and are the following (see Bunning 2004, p. 18 for details):

- Developing and enhancing communication
- Developing and supporting autonomy
- Promoting health
- Developing and adapting identity
- Identifying barriers and promoting participation.

Clinical reasoning

Although there is a lot of individual 'intuitiveness' in decisions about intervention, these decisions should always be based on the application of scientific principles of reasoning and critical thinking (Andolina 2001). Clinical reasoning is based on a combination of pattern recognition, decision-making trees, collection of all possible data, hypothetical–deductive reasoning (discussed in Chapter 3) and reflection by thinking about your own thinking (McAllister and Rose 2000).

The client

Most importantly, the form that the intervention takes must be negotiated with the client and often several other people who are concerned with his or her care. Both the intervention and the anticipated end result must be first and foremost acceptable to the client and also, as far as possible, meet the objectives of other parties, including significant family members, friends and carers, and other key professionals.

Intervention decisions can be made only according to the knowledge that you have of the client, and hence of his or her needs, at a particular point in time. The process of continuous assessment and evaluation, the assimilation of new knowledge about the client and his or her world, and your perceived and objective awareness of change in the client will lead you to modify your intervention decisions over time. The following examples illustrate this:

- At an initial meeting you may choose to offer rather general information to the client but, at subsequent meetings, as you know more and the client can cope with more details, you are likely gradually and selectively to provide more specific advice.
- At an early session you might test out the likelihood of one or other of two therapy approaches being more successful, before the introduction in future sessions of a full programme of the one that is found to be more suitable.
- You might incorporate a small child into a group to develop listening, attention and general communication skills in readiness for individual therapy at a later date, which concentrates on specific aspects of his language problem.
- As you observe deterioration in a progressive disorder in a person whom you have been helping to maintain some speech intelligibility, the focus of your work may be redirected to facilitating swallowing control and the introduction of communication systems apart from speech.

Even within a single interaction with a client, you can alter your tack as new evidence and behaviours emerge. Thus, you might abandon a planned activity to encourage spoken language because the client expresses an immediate need and preference that day for guidance to improve writing to fill in forms, or discloses concerns relating to the communication problem that needs addressing through counselling. In this way, intervention and the range of strategies introduced are tailor-made and flexibly applied in response to the shifting needs of the individual client.

Although intervention decisions are founded on your own knowledge, experience and beliefs and, as discussed above, on the needs and wishes of the people concerned, other vital influencing factors must not be ignored. In particular, as discussed in Chapter 1, you will need to consider the extent and quality of resources available and ensure that the provision offered is equitable, i.e. takes full account of the needs of all potential clients. Numerous questions have to be answered to guide your decisions. Does your service have the staff to enable you to offer individual intensive treatment over several weeks? Do you have the appropriate specialist skills in dysphagia, child language or bilingual language that are required? Do you have the right space for a group to meet? Do the costs and benefits of domiciliary visits outweigh those of clinic-based treatment? Is it ethical to introduce a client to a computer-assisted system of communication if there is not one available for home use? Should you spend several hours in the working week with one client when there are others receiving less of your attention or still waiting to be seen for an initial appointment? In conclusion, what you would like to offer and what you are able to offer are often in conflict, and decisions may have to be tinged with compromise.

Intervention and change

Intervention is the mechanism by which change takes place. To understand the relationship between intervention and change, it is important to appreciate that any response to intervention is dependent on the person's readiness to change, the progress he or she has already made in achieving change, and on whether the intervention strategy or therapy you have selected is appropriate to facilitate the intended change. You will find that different therapies are introduced according to the stage of change that has been reached, as well as recognition of the specific subsequent changes that you perceive are needed.

The starting point for change is an agreement between the client and clinician that something needs to alter. Knowing the change(s) that you wish to bring about, the individual circumstances and the client's current level of readiness to change, you will draw on the many possible approaches that could be used and select the intervention strategies that fit best. Following this pattern, the comprehensive model of change described by Prochaska and DiClemente (1986) stresses that change involves more than a response to intervention applied at one point in time. It depends on the readiness of the client to respond over time within a cycle of stages of change: from 'precontemplation' to 'contemplation', then 'action' and finally 'maintenance'. The authors also stress the importance of accepting that relapse is part of the cycle and of supporting clients through this and back onto the cycle of change once again.

The stages of change are just one aspect of this three-dimensional model. Certain feelings, behaviours and attitudes are engaged during change and these processes will affect the decisions about what techniques and procedures will be of help to this particular client at this particular stage of change. As well as stages and processes, change can take place at different levels. There may be symptom change or cognitive change, or there may be change in interpersonal or family relationships. Change can also affect the inner sense of being or self of the client. Prochaska and DiClemente (1986) point out the importance of the clinician working at the stage/process/level that reflects the needs of the client in order for intervention to be successful. Thus, if a client wishes to discuss and think about his or her difficulty (being at the contemplation stage) and the clinician gives a series of exercises (at the action stage), it is likely that the client will be disinclined to cooperate. Culture can play a big part in the stage at which an individual or family operates. It is vital that the clinician is aware of and sensitive to the cultural expectations for therapy and change. Cultural perceptions of illness, disability and difference will have a strong influence on expectations about what can be done and what can change, as well as the roles of the clinician and the clients in bringing about change (Isaac 2002).

The following definitions and case examples illustrate the components of the stages of change within this model.

Pre-contemplation

At this stage the client will not have acknowledged that a disorder exists, or that change is possible, and so will not have begun to explore his or her condition:

- In a young girl with a language delay referred by a health visitor, this stage may be represented by the mother. The mother may not have recognized that the child is having difficulties, may not have discussed her language behaviours even with those close to her, and may not have sought information to learn more about language development and how to help her daughter.
- A woman who self-refers because she is receiving constant comments about her voice and is being asked if she has a sore throat may not have faced up to the reality of the problem, or the possibility that change could be achieved.

Contemplation

At this stage the client will appreciate that there is a problem and will begin to explore the implications of change and the extent of change, if any, that he or she wishes to make, as well as the methods for change that are available:

- A young man who stutters may be ready to re-evaluate his feelings about his speech and associated behaviours, and about his own identity, and to weigh up whether a proposed change is in his interest.
- A gentleman without voice, after a laryngectomy, may be facing up to a future without conventional speech and considering the options available – oesophageal voice, surgical prosthetic speech rehabilitation or artificial larynges – and the effects of these on his self-image and his communication needs.

Action

At this stage, the client will have negotiated a course of change with the clinician, and strategies will be introduced to effect this change. Also, during this stage, the client should become empowered as changes in behaviour or attitude are shaped:

- A boy with a phonological disorder may be provided with intervention involving listening to sound and word contrasts, and receiving rewards for correct recognition. At the same time the clinician may be providing positive reinforcement when he spontaneously produces correct sounds in conversation, as well as guiding the parents to extend this practice to the home environment. Meanwhile, the child's learning and success during this stage help him to learn that he has the power to manage change.
- A girl who is speechless may be systematically taught to use an electronic communicator, learning the meaning and location of symbols, and the means to select symbols to convey messages. Eventually, with appropriate support and encouragement, the child may begin to use the device creatively to send spontaneous messages, thus relinquishing his or her dependence on the clinician.

Maintenance

At this stage change will have been demonstrated, but support is needed for it to be fully established in the client's everyday life and to enable him or her to face novel situations and people whom he or she has not previously encountered with the changed behaviours and feelings:

- A man who has aphasia and has shown change in language behaviours, developed strategies to cope with a range of communication situations and come to terms with his condition will need continued support as he begins to return to work or engage in new social contexts. Group therapy, simulations of real-life communication exchanges and therapy sessions to discuss experiences when he first re-enters old, or encounters new, social situations might be made available. In this way, opportunities are provided for him to assess whether he is making maximal use of his coping mechanisms and to monitor his acceptance of himself, and to reduce the likelihood of regression.
- A woman who has shown steady voice recovery after episodes of intermittent dysphonia may be seen again after a break of several weeks to discuss factors influencing any setbacks and whether she is satisfied with the changes made.

After satisfactory progress of change(s) through to maintenance, the clinician is likely to terminate her involvement with the client. It is important to point out here that in practice, and for a variety of reasons, intervention can be terminated at earlier stages. Once the client has left therapy, it is important for him or her to be aware of the possibility of relapse, a further to-be-expected stage in the Prochaska and DiClemente (1986) model, and of ways and means both to accept and/or counteract this aspect of the cycle of change.

Readiness to change is not merely a matter of being provided with strategies that will promote change, but also depends on factors such as physical and cognitive development, environmental influences and experiential opportunities. The contribution of these factors informs our clinical knowledge, e.g.:

- A child with phonological delay cannot be expected to acquire a more sophisticated use of speech sounds before attaining an appropriate level of physiological and cognitive maturation.
- Improvement in the language use of an adult with aphasia is in large part the result of the degree of neurophysiological recovery.
- The therapy response of a person with a voice disorder may be dependent on alterations in the environment, such as a reduction in exposure to noise, stress and pollution.
- A child with a language delay can respond maximally to therapy only if the environment provides the right experience and encouragement.

The speech and language clinician takes these factors into account and works with them to the best advantage for the client.

Intervention for prevention or maintenance

Some children, because of physical or psychological traumas or environmental deprivation, may be at risk of failing to develop speech and language or fluency abilities that will enable them to progress in life. These children and their families may need support, education, advice and resources that may be provided by a team of professionals or an individual.

John's father has a stammer which he feels has held him back in his life and work. John is now 2 years old and his parents are very anxious that the stammer may emerge in his speech soon. The speech and language clinician can be both realistic by acknowledging that stammering does occur in families, but also positive in identifying a number of ways in which John's mother and father can reduce the environmental factors that may exacerbate any dysfluency that John may have in his speech.

Sally is worried about her baby who is not thriving very well. Sally is a lone mother struggling with problems of finance, housing and abusive relationships. She and others like her are attending a parent information and support group which is run by a number of professionals including a speech and language therapist. The group has been set up at a Sure Start Children's Centre with money and guidelines provided by the UK government as part of an initiative to provide support to disadvantaged communities and thus reduce risk of longer-term problems (www.surestart.gov.uk).

Annie is being seen at the child development centre in a city hospital. She had a very difficult birth and was very premature. She is now 12 months old and is being monitored by a number of professionals including the speech and language clinician. Annie's parents have needed help in feeding her in the early stages and now Annie is being helped to chew more effectively. The speech and language clinician is also carefully observing and recording Annie's babbling and early words, and is advising her parents on games that will encourage her to listen and to enjoy producing speech sounds.

A number of people may have completed therapy but may be at risk of relapse. These individuals may receive some form of intervention to reduce the chance of relapse. This may be regular but well-spaced visits to the speech and language clinic. It may be that the clinician has arranged for the individual to attend a self-help group, or there may be a volunteer visiting provided by an organization such as Dysphasic Support (Stroke Association at www.stroke.org.uk).

Intervention for rehabilitation or development

You will find that the readiness to change, and the motivations and aspirations, are different for each client, and in part may vary as a consequence of the nature of the disorder and whether it is developmental or acquired. In recognition of this fact, speech and language intervention is often encapsulated within either a development or, for acquired disorders, a rehabilitation framework.

Rehabilitation

An active process that aims for a person to regain his or her former ability or, where this is not possible, to reach his or her optimum physical, mental, social and vocational capacity, and to be integrated maximally into the environment.

People who have acquired an organically or non-organically related voice disorder, dysarthria, aphasia or some other speech and language disorder such as might present in dementia, psychiatric disorder or head injury, fall into this arena. In some cases the problem may be degenerative and follow a progressive course of deterioration.

Unless cognitive deficits have affected awareness and perceptions (such as in dementia, other acquired psychiatric disorders and in some people after a head injury), people with an acquired communication problem will have a clear knowledge of, and memory for, the experience of their prior speech and language function. Generally, they will want to re-attain this ability, their experience of and belief in what constitutes 'normal' communication. Unfortunately, it is common for clinicians to have to help clients come to terms with the fact that they cannot fully regain their prior communication skills.

Rehabilitation sets out to guide the client towards a new and realistic percept of normalcy, draws on a knowledge of the client's communication status and a range of other areas at the time of the onset of the disorder, and supports the client, through direct and indirect intervention, to attain the best possible outcome. In people with progressive disorders, the goals of rehabilitation will be similarly concerned with making positive change, but will at the same time have to pay particular attention to maintaining change, and will be altered to accommodate the changes that result from the deterioration in the condition.

Development

> The lifelong, continuing and chronologically related process of physical, perceptual, cognitive, personality and social change. Intervention actively aims for the person to enhance and maximally attain his or her potential for development.

Communication disorders in children, whether congenital or acquired in childhood, e.g. developmental dysarthria, developmental language disorder, childhood non-fluency and childhood voice disorders, immediately spring to mind as requiring intervention that addresses development. In addition, adults with learning difficulties or who stutter are often viewed as best served within the sphere of developmental approaches.

Although the parents of children with developmental disorders, and the child in cases where the disorder has been acquired later in childhood, will have some experience and perception of normal development, the client will not have a knowledge of communication functioning other than that which they have already achieved. The motivation of the client may be, for example, to enjoy the immediate experience of intervention, to minimize the distress caused to him or her by others, or to help him or her to achieve what peers are achieving. Except perhaps in the case of acquired childhood disorders, and these are not very common, children will not be striving to revisit a previous level of achievement in the continuum of development. Intervention will consider the stage of development already achieved and the future stages that the person should be able to experience, and how to encourage the person to progress.

In conclusion, among the many factors that influence intervention decisions there are certain differences in acquired and developmental disorders, in particular related to experience, potential, motivation and expectations. Once again, you will have to draw on a comprehensive knowledge of intervention theory and approaches and apply the strategies that best meet the client's requirements.

Models of intervention

The importance of providing intervention that is varied and flexible to meet the needs of the individual client has already been highlighted. Not surprisingly there is a wealth of approaches that the speech and language clinician can draw on and apply in diverse ways when responding to the wide-ranging and ever-changing needs of the client within an individual, client-centred holistic management programme. Current models of health professional practice drive our thinking and decisions about intervention. The following are examples of these.

A model of the professional as an 'interactor'

In this model the professional liaises with others and interacts with the environment pertinent to the client (Higgs and Jones 2000). This model is similar to that proposed by an environmental systems theory (Lubinski 1994) which highlights the reliance of any one part of a system on any other for its effective working.

For example, in a factory, the elements of the system might include the production units, the computer and information systems section, the administration department, the despatch centre, the marketing department, the sales staff, and so on, which in turn have a variety of links with external agencies. If a machine in the factory breaks down, it will not just affect the supply of completed items for the next stage in the production line. It may also necessitate reports to, and investigations by, the safety regulators, cause groups of managers to wrestle with balance sheets that reflect losses, require examination by maintenance personnel, involve planners in meetings to decide whether a replacement machine is needed, and so on, engaging numerous elements of the system. In addition, the external environment will be drawn in, perhaps because customers complain when they fail to receive goods on time, or machinery manufacturers are approached to supply an updated machine.

Now let us look more closely at this model in terms of human systems and the individual who has a communication problem. Each individual is the core of a system and possesses his or her own set of characteristics or elements, such as educational, socioeconomic and occupational status, sex, age and race, and physical, emotional and psychological characteristics, such as blue eyes, short-sightedness, screeching laugh, outgoing personality, anxiety or creativity. Many of these characteristics shift and change to a greater or lesser degree in the course of time. Thus, if a person loses his or her sight, he or she may become more dependent on others or may adapt his or her existing interests, e.g. the person may start to use Braille cards to play bridge, develop new interests that are less reliant on vision, use touch and listening to orient him- or herself, need more time to complete tasks, experience episodes of frustration and depression, and walk with less certainty. It is the interaction of all the characteristics that affects the way the individual looks, feels and behaves. It is also these characteristics that are central in influencing how the individual will participate as a member of the environmental system beyond.

This wider environmental system of networks of relationships with other people and the physical world can be separated into (Lubinski 1994):

- a primary system: the family and extended family (e.g. a child living with a single parent, a widow living alone, a married couple living with two children whereas a third child lives independently from them, two men or women living in a partnership)
- a secondary system: an extended environmental system, consisting of:
  - the places and things of the physical environment (e.g. buildings, theatres, railway stations, tin openers, scissors, telephones, computers)
  - the sociocultural environment of customs, values and standards of various groups, such as churches, schools, workplaces or groups such as walking clubs, women's organizations or therapy groups
  - the economic resources available that influence the ability to access opportunities.

A communication disorder, whether caused by repaired cleft palate, a developmental speech disorder or an acquired aphasia, constitutes one of the elements or characteristics of the individual. It will influence the way the person looks, feels and behaves, and also how he or she functions in the environment and how the environment responds to him or her. You could illustrate this with any case you have met in the clinic. Here is just one example.

Pete

A 19 year old who was unemployed, lived with his parents and three younger sisters, and enjoyed lively pub outings with a gang of friends, suddenly developed swallowing difficulties and dysarthria. He had to adopt a pattern of head tilting when drinking, and closing his jaw and holding his lips together for eating. He was anxious about the sound of his speech and irritated by having to repeat much of what he said. The only way to avoid having to repeat himself was to modify the length and complexity of what he said and he felt that this was taking away his natural flow and something of his personality. Outwardly, he did not show that he minded the problem and he began to behave in outrageous ways, such as driving carelessly or playing pranks, which raised a laugh and helped him retain a place within his group of friends. His speech was most difficult to follow when there was a noisy background, such as when the television was on, in the pub, or when competing against the banter of his friends in the car. His friends did not wait while he took a turn in conversation and his family was embarrassed for him, but unsure how to help, so did everything possible to minimize what he had to say.

As already stressed, a speech and language clinician must look beyond the observed features or characteristics of the disorder. You must ensure that you provide comprehensive communication therapy and, to do this, intervention has to consider three perspectives:

1. Ways to help the client adapt, emotionally as well as in functional terms, to the impact of the disorder.
2. Ways to help the family and other significant people in the client's life to cope positively and maximally develop their communicative effectiveness with the individual.
3. Ways to reduce the barriers to communication and increase the opportunities for communication for the individual in the environment at large.

The following are some examples of different types of intervention introduced to address each of these perspectives of Pete's system.

1. The client:
   - Dysphagia therapy: analyse the swallowing pattern in drinking and eating contexts. Encourage drinking of iced water between mouthfuls. Reinforce the use of already adopted and current and new compensatory patterns.
   - Dysarthria therapy: analyse the positive and negative factors affecting intelligibility. Concentrate on phrasing and the articulation of sounds in phrases and sentences. Encourage pauses for swallowing and taking breath, providing feedback on performance. Introduce gradually less structured contexts where the content was unfamiliar to the clinician.
   - Support and guidance: listen to Pete's concerns. Identify his positive characteristics, share ideas about why he feels people are reacting in certain ways and search for possible alternatives and solutions.
   - Incorporate family and friends in discussion and practice sessions with Pete and the clinician in either clinic or home settings (see point 2 below).
   - Liaise with the person who referred Pete, the consultant neurologist and his GP to advise them of the speech and language management and the progress made, and to learn more of the nature of the medical condition and other factors that would inform future intervention decisions.
2. The family and extended family:
   - Through Pete, arrange for one of his mates to come with him to a speech and language therapy clinic to talk about what is involved in communication in general. Create the opportunity for Pete and his friend to express their views on each other's behaviours and consider ways to improve their communication participation.
   - Arrange a visit to Pete at home following similar principles to those of the meeting(s) with his friends, but also to give explanations of the swallowing and speech problems. Guide them, through discussion and practice, to work with him, giving positive feedback on his performance, improving their participation in communication with Pete, and identify factors and opportunities that will benefit him.

3. The physical, sociocultural and economic environment:
    *   Support Pete in introducing himself to Social Services and voluntary organizations to seek new openings for social and work contacts and opportunities for communication that could raise his self-esteem. Encourage him to ensure that he receives maximal financial and other support so that he can access as wide a range of opportunities as possible.
    *   Advise Pete and his family about positive and negative environments for speech, such as switching off background sound before engaging in conversation and making sure that the listener is facing him to gain information from visual messages rather than relying on the auditory messages of his speech that are often unintelligible.

The important thing to remember is the interconnectedness of all aspects of the system and the fact that any intervention will have an impact on the whole system, not just on the individual.

Social–ecology model or social–interactionist model

Another model of health care that informs intervention is the social-ecology model or social–interactionist model (Brechin 1999). The health service has adopted a social model and moved away from the medical model in its planning and decision-making about health issues. The social–interactionist model focuses on both the individual and the social world, and directs intervention at people's ability to function within their social setting. This is the model used in initiatives such as Sure Start (www.surestart.gov.uk), where the speech and language clinician will be one of a team who go out into the community and learn about its cultural values and needs and engage with members of the community to empower them to develop and improve their situation themselves.

World Health Organization framework

The World Health Organization (WHO 2001) framework is an international classification of functioning, disability and health that is based on three components: body structures and functions (impairment), activity limitation and participation restriction. Enderby (1992) added a fourth aspect to the original 1980 WHO system (impairment, disability and handicap) which was 'distress'. These categories are useful for helping you make clinical decisions about the severity of the difficulty and/or the focus of intervention. They also encourage a holistic view of the client and prevent exclusive focus on the impairment, which can sometimes exacerbate rather than improve the condition. Definitions of the terms and examples are given below.

Body function and structure (impairment)

Any loss or abnormality of anatomical, physiological or neurological structure or function.

Examples of this impairment are: migraine, autism, a broken arm, Parkinson's disease, dementia, phonological disorder, dysarthria and a pragmatic language disorder.

Activity limitation (disability)

Any restriction or lack, resulting from an impairment, of ability to perform an activity in the manner or within the range considered normal.

Examples are an inability, reduction or abnormality in dressing, eating, reading, writing, communicating or interacting with others.

Participation restrictions (handicap)

A disadvantage for a given individual, resulting from an impairment or disability, that limits or prevents the fulfilment of a role, depending on age, sex and social/cultural factors, for that individual.

Examples are lack of fulfilment of potential, poor self-esteem, dependence on others, lack of confidence.

Distress

The negative emotional response of the individual or others as a consequence of the impairment, the activity limitation or the participation restriction.

By considering all these aspects relating to a communication or swallowing disorder, the speech and language clinician will be drawn into designing an intervention programme that goes beyond the impairment and addresses the emotional and functional needs of the client. An example is given below.

Tina

Tina is a 5 year old with a severe phonological disorder, who was largely unintelligible to her peers, family and teachers. Her hearing, motor and cognitive development was within the normal range for her age. She lived at home with an older sister and parents, who were all very protective of her. At home and school she avoided speaking situations and presented as a shy and solitary child. She was subject to teasing by the other children in the class. The teacher was aware of Tina's potential ability in comprehension, number, drawing and copying, but, as a result of difficulties in readily understanding what Tina was saying, avoided speech exchange with her and so did not encourage Tina to express ideas. Tina often complained of being unwell before school and her attendance and educational progress were causing increasing concern.

The four perspectives of the intervention are:

1. Intervention directed at the functional impairment, i.e. the phonological disorder: games to increase Tina's awareness of the differences between widely dissimilar sounds, and also games to help her link specific sounds (e.g. /s/ and /t/) with word meanings (e.g. /see/ and /tea/).
2. Intervention directed at the activity limitation, i.e. not expressing ideas, poor educational progress: introduction of signing and picture pointing to support her unintelligible speech so that Tina can offer ideas and the teacher can recognize her abilities.
3. Intervention offered at the level or participation restriction, i.e. Tina's shyness and her avoidance of speaking situations (same as already there).
4. Intervention for the distress, i.e. Tina's obvious worry and withdrawal and her parents' anxiety about her poor school performance:
   – encouragement of teachers to create opportunities for her to recognize her successes in non-speech activities
   – encouragement of parents to praise Tina more and to enrol her (if she wishes) in activities in which she can excel, such as dancing
   – for the clinician to be a listening ear for the parents' concerns and to act as liaison between home and school.

As can be seen from the above cases and discussion, intervention can be applied in infinite ways.

Intervention approaches

The speech and language clinician will identify and describe the specific intervention strategies that have been selected for a particular client (e.g. liaison with parents, teaching specific language programmes, teaching methods to introduce a particular system of communication, reinforcing positive communication attempts, discussing coping strategies, contributing to team meetings with other professionals). At the same time, each strategy will generally be explained in broad terms that can be categorized using the following headings:

• Direct and indirect
• Individual and group
• Intensive and non-intensive.

A variety of combinations of these approaches may figure in the management of clients. One individual with a communication disorder might be engaged in individual, direct and non-intensive therapy, whereas another might experience group, direct and intensive therapy. In addition, as seen in the previous discussion, a client may be involved in different combinations of types of intervention at various times over their contact with the speech and language clinician. Even within a single day, the clinician may be guiding both direct and indirect approaches in the interest of the client, whereas the client may be spending time in both individual and group therapy. The scope of these approaches will be made clearer from the following more detailed discussion of each term.

Direct model of intervention

Direct intervention involves the client, or a group of clients, and the clinician in a face-to-face relationship. It does not mean that the intervention is directive or didactic. Far from this, very often the approach taken is non-directive, the clinician taking the lead from the client rather than instructing the client(s) in what they should do, e.g. Allen (1992) and Hubbell (1981) both describe how the clinician responds to, rather than controls, the behaviour of language-disordered children. However, more directive approaches are also encompassed in direct intervention. The operant conditioning approaches to stuttering in young children (Onslow 1992, Costello 1993) and motor programming therapies for acquired speech apraxia (Wertz et al. 1984, Square-Storer 1989, Miller and Docherty 1995) are examples of more directive methods used in direct intervention. Very often a combination of methods with varying degrees of directive, or instructive, and non-directive strategies will be incorporated.

The essential feature is that the client, or clients, and clinician are physically together in the interaction. In addition, parents, carers, teachers or others involved in the management programme may be present. The following are all examples of direct intervention:

- Guidance in the use of computers and assistive systems of communication
- Teaching sign language
- Counselling
- Exercises to enhance listening and comprehension abilities
- Therapy, involving modelling, shaping and reinforcement to encourage greater effectiveness in the use of sounds, words, grammar or other communication behaviour, lends itself to direct methods of intervention.

Even when this face-to-face mode of intervention figures prominently in a management programme, the speech and language clinician may be orchestrating simultaneous indirect intervention.

Indirect model of intervention

Indirect intervention encompasses all those aspects of intervention that happen outside the face-to-face, client or client group interaction with the clinician. Examples of indirect intervention include:

- Designing programmes that are explained to and then implemented by teachers, nursing staff, carers, volunteers, parents and other significant communication partners of a client or group of clients, so that learning and change can take place in contexts where the clinician is not present.
- Consultation, by asking, informing, advising, conferring and reporting about a client or client group in order to contribute to the management decisions that other professionals are making, to guide the speech and language management decisions of the clinician, and to seek resources for the client or client group.
- Consultation with relatives and other significant people in the lives of individuals with communication disorders to learn more about the background of the client, and the concerns, reactions and understandings of these people known to the client, and to give support, explanations and advice that will benefit the client.
- Setting up of support groups for carer and client groups.
- Promoting awareness of communication disorder and the service provided by speech and language clinicians, and encouraging referral and access to the service for people with communication problems.
- Promoting an understanding of communication disorder, non-discriminatory attitudes and behaviours towards people with communication disorder, and factors that exacerbate or prevent problems associated with communication disorder.
- Initiating training for volunteers, professionals or other carers to improve their understanding about particular client groups, and to maximize the communication effectiveness of their interactions with the client group.

More about all these aspects of indirect intervention are covered later in the book.

Individual therapy model of intervention

Individual, or one-to-one, therapy is often called 'traditional therapy' and is sometimes scorned as being unimaginative and failing to reflect the communicative environment of the real world. However, not only is a one-to-one interaction the most common context for language use, it is also the most common context for language learning from the cradle onwards. As in all intervention, if it is assessed to be the most appropriate type to meet the needs of the client at a particular point in time, every effort should be made to respond to this judgement.

This type of intervention concentrates on a single client. The clinical intervention may be direct or indirect and may involve several others with a part to play in working with the client towards altering communication and attitudes. Teachers, parents, carers, helpers and other professionals may be incorporated into the therapy, either actively or passively, so that they can observe, be consulted, advised or counselled. The client may be introduced to specific speech and language learning, and coping strategies, or provided with opportunities to explore communicative achievements, but always in the absence of other clients. Some of the characteristics of individual intervention are as follows:

- It provides intervention that is tailor-made for one client, and this can be modified solely to meet the shifting needs of that client.
- It can simulate the one-to-one communication partnerships that commonly occur in everyday life.
- It can be facilitative or didactic, depending on the therapy methods that are applied.
- It protects the client from interruption, sidetracking or inhibition by other clients. Maximal time is given to the interests of the client.
- Its intensity can be threatening for some clients, whereas other clients find this type of intervention significantly less threatening than a group context.

Group therapy model of intervention

Group treatment is merely the treatment of more than one client in the same session (Davis and Wilcox 1985). The purposes and methods employed can be vastly different, but an essential component is that by bringing two or more people together you have created a social unit in which the participants have a face-to-face interaction (Sears et al. 1988). The client is not confined to interactions with the clinician and any other attendant person concentrating solely on his or her own case, but participates in therapy related to the needs, concerns and behaviours of other clients too.

When forming a group, important decisions have to be made about its size, membership, structure and objectives. You have to remember that if the group is over-large there could be inadequate opportunities for maximal involvement of all participants. If it is too small, some members may feel intimidated. As long as each member can achieve personal objectives within the group experience, and there are also some mutually acceptable objectives, members need not have common features in terms of such things as background and type and severity of communication disorder. Thus, a communication group might consist of people with dysarthria, aphasia and mild dementia, with various experiences of therapy, who have dissimilar educational, work experience, social backgrounds and interests. Remember, in social settings, that people with diverse experiences and characteristics meet in groups. If your primary intention is to develop communication skills within a social context, a heterogeneous group should not be discounted.

You will know from personal experiences of being in a group of people, e.g. a social club, committee, colleagues, family or children at play, that individuals take on particular roles, whether by formal or informal means, and relate to each other in different ways. Not surprisingly, when participants either join or leave the group there are shifts of roles and behaviours, i.e. the dynamics of the group, and even the sense of direction for the group, change. In recognition of these features of group interaction, the speech and language clinician will make a decision as to whether an 'open' or 'closed' group is appropriate to achieve the objectives set. An open group tends to have greater flexibility and formality, and fewer clear definitions of structure and objectives, than a closed group.

An example of an open group would be a support group for people with aphasia, where newcomers are welcome and existing members attend with or without carers, if and when they choose, the purpose being to practise communication skills, gain confidence through experimentation and share experiences with others in a safe environment, which at the same time simulates many aspects of the real world.

An example of a closed group would be for a group for teenagers who stutter that is run on five consecutive days, applying a programme of therapy adopting the principles of avoidance reduction therapy (Sheehan 1975) and block modification (Van Riper 1973; see also Lawson et al. 1993).

A large proportion of the groups formed by speech and language clinicians is both psychotherapeutic and task oriented (Fawcus 1992). The psychotherapeutic aspects provide opportunities to support the psychosocial needs of the participants, such as increasing confidence in communicating, sharing concerns and experiences, responding to disclosures relating to the communication difficulty, and practising speech and language skills in a more natural setting. The task-oriented aspects provide more specific opportunities to improve, e.g. fluency, listening and turn-taking, articulation, grammar and the use of non-speech channels, such as drawing, gesture and pointing to convey messages.

In addition to groups incorporating the client, groups can also be formed for parents, other relatives, friends or carers. Gibbard (1994) gives an example of a parental training group that was held once a fortnight over a 6-month period. Objectives were set for the parents and they were given suggestions of games and methods that they could use to help their child and to help transfer the linguistic learning gained from the activities to everyday situations. The parents discussed and planned together, as well as being guided by the clinician.

It is important to acknowledge that just because people are brought together does not mean that they will instantly constitute an effective group. Participants will need time to become familiar with each other and gain each other's trust, and to understand the methods and objectives of the group. The speech and language clinician has to help the group form, providing opportunities for members to learn something about each other, to appreciate the expectations of the various participants and the purpose of their meeting together, and to clarify the role that the clinician will take. Whitaker (1989) describes this initial stage of the group process as formative and the subsequent stage of ongoing interaction as established. This reflects our earlier discussion of the pre-contemplative, contemplative action and maintenance cycle of change (Prochaska and DiClemente 1986).

An important aspect of groups that must not be neglected is that not only must we facilitate the group forming and achieving its purpose through the established stage, we must also prepare the members for the final, or termination, stage (Whitaker 1989). Many groups will need easing very carefully into the break-up of the support and relationships that they have shared. This preparation for termination applies to both group therapy and individual therapy. For both settings we need to spend time with the client(s) reviewing what has been achieved and coming to terms with a new phase.

Intensive and non-intensive models of intervention

Clinicians vary in their understanding of what constitutes intensive rather than non-intensive intervention. This is largely the result of the individual experience of clinicians and their interpretations of the quantitative and qualitative factors that explain the terms. It is hoped that the following discussion will help formulate an appreciation of these concepts.

The simplest way to think of intensity is in terms of the amount of face-to-face contact time that is concentrated on a client within a given period of weeks or months, i.e. the quantitative, e.g. an hour-long session of group or individual direct therapy each week, even running over several months, is not generally perceived to be intensive. On the other hand, a half-hour session provided several times a week for 2 or 3 weeks is likely to be referred to as intensive. In part, interpretation is based on custom and practice. Some clinicians may consider more than three sessions a week to be intensive, particularly where they commonly see clients for no more than a single session each week.

In determining whether therapy is intensive or non-intensive we must also consider the nature of the clinical contact, i.e. the qualitative value. Although three individual half-hour sessions of therapy across a week might be described as intensive, a 2-hour group session once a week is unlikely to be considered as such, in spite of the longer time in therapy. Further, where therapy is more structured and directed, intervention is more likely to be perceived as intensive, e.g. in the case of a person admitted to a ward with dysphagia, whom we see briefly but daily, we are more likely to describe the intervention as intensive if the contact involves the introduction of a specific programme of dysphagia rehabilitation, rather than simply monitoring progress and readiness for more direct intervention.

As already indicated, intensive and non-intensive intervention are equated with amounts of face-to-face contact time. For every person receiving intensive or non-intensive intervention, a significant amount of time will also be spent on indirect intervention during the same period. We may make three phone calls, write a report, visit a school, attend a case conference, discuss progress and offer advice to parents outside of a weekly therapy session with a small child, but these activities would not be taken into account in determining whether intervention was intensive or non-intensive. It is also important to note that it may not be the speech and language clinician who is responsible for the delivery of intensive therapy. This would be the case where an assistant, teacher or parent is following a concentrated therapy programme under the guidance of the clinician.

The greater our experience of different types of intervention, the greater will be our appreciation of the scope of their dynamics and the possibilities for change that they offer our clients. In later chapters there is further guidance on specific aspects of intervention.

Chapter 3
Assessment: process and practice

If there is a complex thing that we do not yet understand, we can come to understand it in terms of simpler parts which we do already understand.

Dawkins (1986, p. 11)

Assessment appears to be a very complex area, but if you can take note of what Dawkins says and build up a picture of the whole process bit by bit, you will find that you do understand it and are able to undertake the practice that it involves.

So, let us start by defining the words being used and considering the approaches that you will be taking when assessing an individual with a speech and language disorder.

Process is a sequence of operations undergone to reach a goal (the abstract 'conceptualizing') and *practice* is the course of action or the performance of specific activities (the concrete 'doing'). The nature of assessment is to think and do at the same time, so the action cannot be easily extricated from the consideration; thus the two need to be considered side by side. As you can see from Figure 3.1, the whole process of assessment can be broken down into subsections and this is what you will need to do to decide what procedures are needed at what stage. But the gaining of information from clients is never complete, so the process needs to be thought of as cyclical – each new piece of knowledge feeds both forwards into the next stage of the procedure and backwards, causing potential changes to what you already know about your client.

In the profession of speech and language pathology and therapy, we tend to adhere to a scientific approach. This entails critical thinking and clinical reasoning using both deductive and inductive methods. *Deductive reasoning* means drawing conclusions from the data or information that you have or the ideas or premises that are in front of you. It requires a logical and objective way of working through the issues (Andolina 2001). Formal tests are based on deductive reasoning. *Inductive reasoning* is a process of generation of new ideas from an understanding of the patterns of information that are presented. It therefore allows conclusions to be reached even when the data

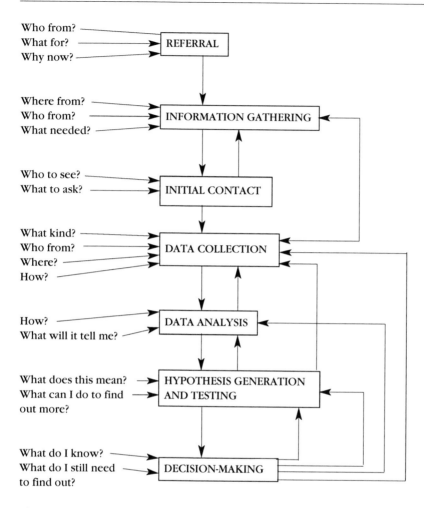

Figure 3.1 A flowchart of the assessment process.

or information are incomplete (Higgs and Jones 2000). An informal assessment approach uses inductive reasoning. *Hypothesis generation*, or the creation of a possible relationship between things, requires both inductive and deductive reasoning 'moving from a set of specific observations to a generalization (inductive reasoning) and moving from a generalization to a conclusion in relation to a specific case (deductive reasoning)' (Higgs and Jones 2000, p. 6). These processes lie at the heart of any competent work in the field of speech and language clinical practice. So, when presented with a client who enters therapy with a particular speech and language problem, you should:

- define the problem
- develop hypotheses
- plan your approach

- consider ways of collecting data
- decide which instruments might be necessary
- decide who is most competent to undertake a particular investigation, e.g. you might wish to take measurements on a laryngograph and need to request this to be done by a colleague in a hospital department that has such equipment
- collect the data
- carefully record the information from contacts with the client or others
- analyse the data
- assemble the information in an orderly fashion
- compare with norms or other criteria if appropriate
- accept or reject the original hypotheses
- generalize from data if appropriate.

Throughout this book, and particularly within this chapter, we ask you to think in an orderly, systematic and therefore scientific way, and to do this we start with a flowchart (see Figure 3.1) to help focus your attention on what you need to do and where you are going during the process of assessment.

Defining assessment

A large part of your role as a speech and language clinician is assessment. You never cease to assess. Through your training you develop the ability to perceive and observe the strengths and weaknesses of your clients' communicative systems (Wirz 1995), as well as your own strengths and weaknesses through reflection (McAllister and Lincoln 2004), and you continue to revise these throughout your contact with a client or group of clients.

Assessment is 'to do with making a judgement about an individual in relation to a large group of people, based on the acquisition of a body of knowledge concerning that individual' (Beech et al. 1993, p. xi). This can be done using either descriptive or prescriptive methods (Wirz 1993). *Descriptive* assessment methods set out to describe in detail the communication behaviour of an individual as a basis for decisions about where problems lie and what might be done about them. *Prescriptive* assessment uses standards or norms as the basis for comparing one person with another. Both forms of assessment involve acquiring a body of knowledge about the particular client and using this as the basis for deciding on a particular course of action.

Before moving on to consider in detail the process defined in Figure 3.1, it is necessary to bear in mind the approaches you might use in assessment. Will your assessment be:

- a screen or a full assessment?
- formal or informal?
- norm-referenced or criterion-referenced?
- standardized or non-standardized?

Screening versus full assessment

Screening is a simplified procedure designed to pick out aspects of behaviour that need to be more fully investigated. In the clinical setting, you may use some play, some matching tasks, some conversation and some problem-solving games with a 4 year old as a general screen of his or her performance. Based on your observations, you may then decide to go ahead with an in-depth assessment of his or her comprehension difficulties, or you may use an already designed screening test, such as the FIRST Screening Test (Fielder 1993), to tap areas of difficulty soon after a client has had a stroke. Once you have a better picture of your client's levels of ability, you may then go ahead with a more comprehensive test battery.

Formal or informal

The division here is between the gathering of information either through some pre-planned, organized or standard procedure, or through an observational approach. A test that can be bought is the most formal procedure that you might use. This would give clear guidelines about administration and would very likely be both standardized and norm-referenced. An example of such a test is the Reynell Developmental Language Scales III (RDLS III – Edwards et al. 1997). A pre-prepared checklist could also be considered a formal procedure. This is likely to be criterion-referenced, such as the Functional Communication Therapy Planner (Worrall 1999). An informal approach would be individualized and consist of observation, recording of behaviour seen and devising appropriate ways of probing more deeply into areas that you feel might be more of a problem for this client. You might start with general conversation with an adult and through this note that there seems to be some lack of intelligibility and slurring of speech. You watch the movements of the client's articulators with care, you note posture and breathing, and you check for spillage during the drinking of a cup of tea. You might also ask this client to imitate certain movements of the articulators or to produce a sound such as [s] or [z] and hold it for as long as possible. Informally, you are building up a picture of this person's difficulties. As you can see, both formal and informal approaches will give valuable information and can be flexibly interwoven in the ongoing process of assessment (see Lees and Urwin 1997, for useful ideas of the formal and informal assessment of children).

Norm-referenced or criterion-referenced

Norm-referenced tests relate the performance of a client to peers of the same age. An example of such a test would be the Clinical Evaluation of Language Functions (CELF-R – Semel et al. 1987) where each subtest can be scored in relation to the ability of children with no language difficulties. The problem of norm-referenced tests in the speech and language area is that it is often inappropriate to relate the performance of many of your clients to a norm.

This is clearly argued by Dockerill and Henry (1993) in relation to adults and children with learning difficulties.

Criterion-referenced assessments give a picture of whether an individual does or does not have a particular skill. A carefully designed scale of this kind is based on a step-by-step breakdown of the behaviours needed for a specified skill, e.g. the Wessex-revised Portage checklist (White and East 1983) gives examples of the language understanding or production to be expected of the child, which can be easily scored as that behaviour is noted. A problem with this type of approach is that individuals do not all conform to a particular order of skill development, so criterion-referenced procedures cannot easily be used to define progress over time.

Standardized or non-standardized

Standardization can be taken to mean a formalized, structured procedure for the administration of a test and/or the carrying out of the test on a sample of people to gain an idea of the range of possible responses to the test items. The more people included in the sample used to standardize a test, the more sure you can be that the behaviours expected by the test are valid, e.g. if you know that the number of side-to-side movements of the tongue expected in 60 seconds is the mean of a large group of adults across a wide age range, you can feel confident that the fact that your client could do only a few movements in that time is significant (see Beech et al. 1993, for lists of tests and the populations on which they were standardized). A non-standardized assessment procedure is no less useful, but for different purposes. Many of the procedures that clinicians use to assess phonology are non-standardized because what is being looked at is the child's unique sound system rather than speech sounds used or not used by others of this age group.

Why assess?

When you first meet a client you will be curious about why he is here, what his difficulty is, how he copes with it and so on. Your professional ethics will push you to understand thoroughly this client's condition in order to make appropriate decisions about his management programme. Your scientific education will constrain you to be cautious and not proceed with therapy until you have a grasp of all the factors that might affect this client's progress. Once your programme of intervention is in place, you will continue to be curious and ask questions, to try to understand more, to use the knowledge that you are gaining to make further decisions. The complexity of this person, with this condition, in this environment, will present on-going and new possibilities for change. So, you assess in order to (Adams et al. 1997, Bunning 2004):

- understand the status of speech, language or swallowing – is there a difficulty?

- make a differential diagnosis
- provide an informed opinion
- help in planning intervention
- provide a baseline from which to measure change
- provide evidence for the choice of intervention
- make decisions about long-term outcomes.

The assessment process

Think of the process of assessment as the fitting together of a jigsaw. You need to find and fit the shapes to form a picture of the person with whom you are to be involved. Unlike the jigsaws that you did as a child (or still do now), you do not have a photograph on the front of the box to guide you. You do, however, have the knowledge gained from the fields of linguistics, psychology, medical sciences, education and sociology as well as your own life knowledge and beliefs, and the client him- or herself – the person who knows what the picture on the front of the box looks like! The assessment process is one of working together to find out as much as possible and to explore as many angles as are appropriate. The theories and ideas from your reading and from your joint investigation can give you confidence in putting the pieces together.

The client in the assessment process

Before we go on to consider each level of the assessment flowchart, it is important to review what has been said before about the word 'client'. Your client may be an individual with a concern, a dyad (mother and child, husband and wife), a family, a carer, a group of carers, a group of professionals or a community. You need to be sensitive to the culture of your clients and how the processes and practices of assessment may impact on their knowledge and beliefs about themselves (Isaac 2002). To simplify the discussion below, we have focused on an individual as the client but we make reference to other service users as appropriate.

Look back at Figure 3.1, the flowchart of the assessment process. We now take time to think about each level of this chart, and the processes and practices it involved: (1) referral; (2) information gathering; (3) the initial contact; (4) data collection; (5) data analysis and evaluation; (6) hypothesis generation and testing; and (7) decision-making: prognosis and priorities.

Referral

Picture yourself in your clinical setting, having just received a letter or a phone call asking you to see a client for the first time. The thrill that you feel – part excitement, part fear – is one felt by even the most experienced clinicians, and it is what makes the work of the speech and language clinician so stimulating. Who will the client be? What problems will he or she bring? How will you go about solving them?

To refer is to hand over something (in this case information on a person) to another. This means that the responsibility for dealing quickly and appropriately with this information is also handed over. The expectation from the referring agent is that you will deal with whatever issues are needed, keep him or her informed and, once you have seen the person or people involved, pass your additional information on to the referrer. The referral may come in the form of a letter, a pre-printed form, a telephone call or a face-to-face contact. Your response must be as speedy as possible, however the information is conveyed. In many work districts, you would be expected to write a letter in response to a referral within a set time (e.g. 1 or 2 weeks).

When you receive a letter from a referring agent you may think 'Can't I refer this person on to . . . who is much better able to deal with this sort of thing?' or 'Can't I discharge this person who has such a minor problem before seeing them?'

No! You have a professional responsibility to assess the situation. Also, the referral letter you have in front of you is the subjective view of the doctor, teacher, social worker, parent, client or whoever the referring agent is. However detailed the information, you still do not know what sort of problems (if any) the person who walks through your door will bring you. It is important that you formulate an objective view of what the problem is, and then you might decide that the best approach is to refer on to a specialist, either one in another field or another speech and language clinician.

Who from?

Referrals may come from a number of sources, from doctors or health visitors, from teachers or professionals working with children in their early years, from Social Services, from colleagues, from the person who has the problem. In some settings an open system will operate where anyone with concerns may come along for an informal discussion. In other settings a more formal process will operate. Different employers may have different views as to from whom you can and cannot receive referrals. Make sure that you know the guidelines for your particular place of work. Also remember that, even if there is a very open referral system, there are still professional courtesies that require you to inform others of your involvement. You will need to thank the referring agent and give an indication of when you hope to make an appointment for the client. Once you have completed your initial investigation of the problem (which may take one or several meetings with the client as well as gathering of information from other sources), you will need to send reports to relevant people (see Chapter 7 for further discussion on report writing).

What for?

Referral letters may contain different amounts of information. Some are very detailed whereas others give only sketchy information about the person you are about to see. The letter may provide you with some clues as to the expectations of the person referring, as well as clues as to what might have already been said by this professional to the client. Look at the letters in Figure 3.2. What might these comments mean about the way in which the referrer views the problem? What do you think the expectations of the referring agent might be of you and your service?

---

1. Referrals from a health visitor:
   'Please see this little girl who cannot say her "s" sounds'.
   or
   'Please see this bright little boy who can't yet talk'.

2. Referrals from a consultant:
   'Please assess and advise Mrs B. following her stroke'.
   or
   'Please could you see this very anxious lady whom I saw in my clinic today and whose vocal cords are completely normal'.

3. Referral from a teacher:
   'John cannot cope with his school work and is becoming a problem because of his speech'.

Figure 3.2 Examples of referral letters.

Why now?

This is a very important question to ask yourself before you see the client, and the client and/or carer, when you have the initial consultation. The referral could be coming to you now because something has happened recently or the pressure to seek help may have been building for some time. Sometimes the referral occurs because of an important event in the client's life. The factors that have instigated the referral are likely to be as much a source of concern as the speech and language difficulty itself and this is why it is so important for you to take account of them. Some of these triggers to referral may be:

- occurrence of a crisis (e.g. a stroke, an imminent laryngectomy)
- perceived interference by the problem with social or personal relationships such as might occur when a person who stutters reaches young adulthood
- pressure by others, e.g. by an employer who finds it difficult to understand the speech of someone who stutters
- persistence of symptoms after a personally set deadline, as might occur when a parent suddenly decides that the child's speech difficulties should have improved by now
- relationship between the problem and other goals (e.g. delayed language in a family with high academic standards)

- access to health-care facilities (e.g. either proximity and/or finance may have made access difficult but this has now changed)
- change in circumstances, e.g. a new manager in a group home who wants her staff to develop additional skills
- a demand from a higher authority, such as the National Service Framework for the Older People (Department of Health or DoH 2001b) where a set of objectives must be met.

Information gathering

Lahey (1988, p. 123) says that 'information should bear directly on identifying whether there is a problem, on determining the goals and procedures for intervention, or on determining progress'. So you do not seek information blindly; you have a plan of what you want to find out and why. Your plan must be constructed carefully, to ensure that nothing is missed. It is your responsibility, once the referral has arrived, to seek out information in a systematic way. A plan is a blueprint for the work to be undertaken. It will consist of aims and objectives as well as the actual procedures that you will undergo to obtain the relevant details. A full discussion of the planning process can be found in Chapter 4.

The way in which you approach the sources of information – by letter, phone or face to face – will influence the type of information that you can obtain. Correct procedures in making contact must be followed. Remember that good communication skills will be essential for the smooth running of information gathering.

Where from and who from?

You will need to seek information from as many sources as possible, indirectly or directly. Indirect sources include:

- hospital notes
- clinic files
- letters from those who know this client
- school reports
- reports from Social Services
- care plans.

You may wish to ask for information directly, in a face-to-face situation, via the telephone or in a written form via letters, e-mails, etc. Some of the people you might contact are listed below, but there will be others whom you may come across. The important thing is to be aware of the need to seek out information that is relevant from as wide a range of sources as possible. Direct sources include:

- client
- parent, spouse or other carer
- other involved people, e.g. friends, community contacts
- referral agent
- relevant consultant
- client's general practitioner
- health visitor or district nurse
- other involved speech and language therapists
- related professionals:
  - physiotherapist
  - occupational therapist
  - social worker
  - clinical psychologist
  - educational psychologist
  - head teacher
  - class teacher
  - managers or staff at Social Services settings, e.g. nurseries, day centres, homes for elderly people, etc.
  - employer.

What is needed?

You must start by considering *why* you need information. You should do this from the perspective of the client and a good way of approaching it is to use the WHO classification mentioned in Chapter 2. As you want to understand the problems from the client's perspective, you need to find out about:

- the impairment (body function and structure)
- medical factors
- developmental factors
- linguistic factors
- cognitive factors
- activity limitation
- the client's ability to communicate
- effects of the problem on education
- effects on work and leisure
- effects on family roles
- participation restriction
- the client's relationships with others
- the client's involvement in the community
- the client's distress/avoidance/withdrawal.

You will need to gather information in all these areas and use of a model or a framework to prompt your memory will be necessary.

The Venn diagram has been used by many authors as a useful tool for demonstrating the overlap between particular aspects of the behaviours under investigation. Lahey (1988) has used a Venn diagram to help us conceptualize language as being composed of the areas of content, form and use which may be seen as discrete but which overlap and merge in a fully functioning system. Also Wall and Myers (1984) have used this diagram to identify particular areas of concern for children who stutter. Another model used in the stuttering literature is that of Rustin et al. (1995), which uses a grid-like framework for identifying areas to investigate.

Figure 3.3 suggests models that you might use. You will need to bulk out these general models with more detail as indicated below. These lists are not conclusive; there will be other factors that you can add as you become aware of them.

Medical information

You may need to consider some or all of the following depending on the problem:

- General health: at present and in the past, how this affects the person and the problem.
- Nature of the disorder, e.g. progressive, acute onset, developmental.
- Neurological factors: evidence of brain damage or neurological dysfunction from the notes.
- Pertinent illnesses: upper respiratory problems or otitis media may have affected hearing, bronchitis may be associated with voice disorder, encephalitis may have led to memory loss, etc.
- Sensory abilities: particularly hearing and vision where the problem may be one of acuity or perception or both.
- Motor abilities: gross or fine motor skills may be different from what might be expected.
- Ways in which medical problems have been dealt with:
  – surgical procedures particularly significant in cleft palate or laryngectomy, glossectomy, etc.
  – drugs, which may well have an impact on the speech and language, memory, articulation of the client (see Vogel and Carter 1995 for useful information on drugs, and speech and language behaviour).
- What is still being treated?
- Which medical professionals are involved?
- Family history: many speech and language conditions are either part of a genetic condition, such as fragile X syndrome, which runs in families, or have a familial tendency, such as stuttering where there is up to a 71 per cent chance that a child who stutters will have a member of the extended family who also stutters (Ambrose et al. 1993).
- Developmental information: the way in which the child has developed over time and the speed of this in relation to expected norms is vital information.

(a)

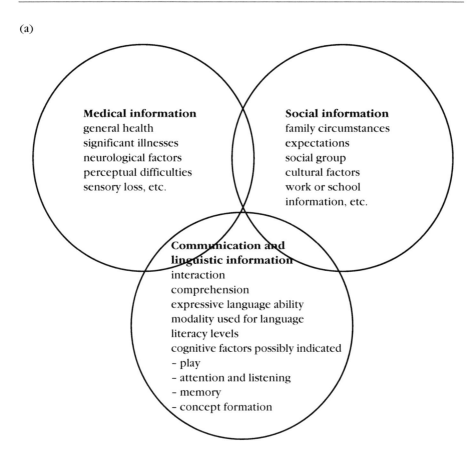

Medical information
general health
significant illnesses
neurological factors
perceptual difficulties
sensory loss, etc.

Social information
family circumstances
expectations
social group
cultural factors
work or school
information, etc.

Communication and
linguistic information
interaction
comprehension
expressive language ability
modality used for language
literacy levels
cognitive factors possibly indicated
- play
- attention and listening
- memory
- concept formation

(b)

Physiological factors	Social/emotional factors
medical information	awareness of problem
hearing and vision	feelings about problem
motor control	relationships
family history	emotional stability
developmental details	social skills

Environmental factors	Cognitive factors
family circumstances	language
school/work information	play
pressure from others	attention
demands of environment	memory
reaction of others to problem	learning ability

Figure 3.3 Information gathering models: (a) a Venn diagram (after Wall and Myers, 1984, p. 7); (b) a grid model (after Rustin et al., 1995, p. 38)

You will also be interested in the long-term developmental course of disorders such as cleft palate, stuttering, cerebral palsy, etc., because this will give you a view on positive or negative changes over time. Being alert to change over time will allow you to chart the progress of neurological disorders such as motor neuron disease or take account of the changes found in dementia neurone.

Creating a developmental profile

It is essential that you become competent at identifying differences from normative development in the children whom you see. To do this, you might make, as a clinical tool, a developmental profile in an easy-to-carry folder or on file cards. Your profile should cover a fairly wide age range, from birth to 5 years for all aspects, and then from 5 years to adolescence for specific language skills (e.g. the ability to make inferences or tell or understand jokes), or problem-solving and abstract thinking. The following areas are suggested:

• Physical growth including such things as head circumference
• Reflexes
• Gross motor development
• Fine motor development
• Perceptual abilities
• Social/moral development
• Cognitive development
• Concept development and learning levels
• Development of play
• Language development.

Information is available from books, videos, developmental charts, lecture notes and experience in clinic and of children in other settings. The file will need to be added to as your knowledge grows and you should cross-reference to make sure that you are gaining a full picture. Figure 3.4 shows examples of developmental profile entries.

To help you make use of the knowledge you are gathering, you must draw on your understanding of theory concerning the relationship between certain traumas, diseases, genetic conditions, drug doses, sensory loss, developmental delay, etc., and behaviour including language and speech (Table 3.1).

Social/emotional and environmental information

There are numerous areas that can be considered under this heading. The following are some of the more common factors that may well have significance in helping you to understand the speech and language difficulties of your clients:

You may wish to have your entries identified by behaviour:

> **Social behaviour 2.06 years**
>
> Very active, dislikes restraint
> Little understanding of common danger
> Very dependent on adult

> **Motor development 2.06 years**
>
> Walks upstairs and down confidently but places two feet on each step
> Runs well straight forward
> Climbs easy apparatus

Or you may take an age and identify a range of behaviours within that:

> **Age 2.06 years**
>
> Motor skills: gross motor - walking upstairs and down with ease
> Fine motor - builds tower of seven cubes using preferred hand
> Social skills: unaware of danger very dependent on adult
> Needs parent close by
> Language skills: comprehension - understands large
> vocabulary and SVO, SVA structures
> Expression - asks questions 'what?', 'where?'

Figure 3.4 Examples of developmental profile entries.

- Family circumstances: who is in the family, what are relationships like in the family, how does your client fit into the family structure, what are the support networks for the family, are there any financial or other pressures on the family, what are the language levels in the family, what expectations do they have for the child, what languages occur in the home, what language models are being given?
- Social and cultural factors affecting the family and the client: what expectations are placed on the client for language performance from his or her social grouping or culture, what role does this client play in the social or cultural structures?
- Work and school information: this will give clues as to educational status, interests, environmental factors (noise, pollutants), lifestyle (consistency, stressors, such as time pressure).
- Awareness, self-esteem, expectations of self, etc., will be important in understanding the client's motivation, level of anxiety or depression, etc.
- Leisure and social involvement: this information will give some idea of health, friendships, sociability, group belongingness, etc.

Table 3.1 Examples of the influence of medical factors

Problem	Medical factor
Mrs S has a voice problem	This may be affected by her use of an inhaler
Jane has phonological difficulties	It appears that these are related to intermittent hearing loss during periods of otitis media
David has been in a road traffic accident	His inability to initiate purposive communication may be related to the brain damage he sustained. The drugs used to control the epilepsy which has since developed may also be implicated in his generally slow response to questions
Mr C is unable to obtain reasonable oesophageal voice	This may well be related to his long-term bronchial problems
John has a stutter	Developmental factors which may be significant are both emotional and learning difficulties during his school life
Ann has learning difficulties	Developmental information of significance is the emergence of spoken words at 10 years of age and two and three word combinations at 15 years. Was this just very slow development or were there significant factors occurring at these times?

Your client is a part of a system (Barker 1996). His or her family forms the core of the system; society, school, friends, etc. form a second system, and the client's cultural background forms another larger system. All these systems are interconnected. The slow development, lack of development or loss of speech and language in one individual has implications for the feelings, lifestyle and methods of managing for that individual's significant others. You will need to understand how the family, school or social group from which your client comes is reacting to his or her particular speech and language disorder. You must be particularly careful that you understand the expectations and norms of behaviour linked to the particular culture from which your client comes.

The wider family or social network is very important to consider. Think of yourself and of the people around you. Whom do you rely on for what? Who helps you when you are down? Whom can you have a good laugh with? A person's support system is sorely tried when that person has developed a problem. Many of you will have come across a client who has had a stroke, for example, and who is now visited by very few of his or her previous friends. Your client's ability to cope with whatever has happened and to work for positive change will be related to aspects such as support, the number of losses that he or she has experienced and the amount of life change that has been brought about (Table 3.2).

Table 3.2 Examples of social, emotional and environmental factors

Problem	Social/environmental factors
Mr B has poor speech intelligibility and is unable to write as a result of his Parkinson's disease	Mr B has always been in charge of the family finances and his inability to communicate with his bank is causing both him and Mrs B a great deal of unhappiness at present
Arfan has a developmental language problem	At 4 years of age Arfan is in a nursery setting where English is spoken. At home his family speak Gujerati. Having two languages is putting additional strain on Arfan's immature language skills
Joan has a voice disorder	Joan works as a typist/secretary in an open-plan office. She is often talking on the phone above the noise of machines and people. This may be a factor in the abuse of her voice
Mrs C has dysarthria	Mrs C has no immediate family. A niece visits her and does her shopping weekly. You feel that Mrs C's dysarthria will improve with practice but she speaks to very few people from week to week. The majority of her speaking is done when she comes to see you

Communication, speech and language, swallowing information

Your main aim in the assessment process is to gather relevant information about the abilities and difficulties of your client(s) and about how they impact on the daily lives of these individuals and those around them. Speech and language clinicians are always interested in the person in interaction with others. Communication of any sort is a two-way (or more) process. Within this process there will be a constant shift from the role of giver to that of receiver of information. It is vital therefore for the individual to be competent at:

* receiving the message via the senses
* interpreting the message through the cognitive processes of decoding and making sense of the information
* planning the response through the cognitive processes of encoding and organizing the message in preparation for producing it
* producing the message via the motor system.

(See Crystal and Varley 1998, for a fuller discussion of the communication chain.)

Messages can be passed via the auditory–oral system where the information is spoken and heard, or via the visual–manual system where information is provided through the hands (a signed language). These are the main systems that you might come across, but you will also deal with individuals who require the receipt and passing of messages via a tactile system.

To ensure that you do not forget to notice behaviour in certain areas of communication, you need a framework or plan for your assessment. As already mentioned, the Venn diagram provided by Lahey (1988) is extremely useful. Under her headings of form, content and use, you may think of the following:

- *Form* means the structure of language. An investigation of this area will involve the identification of your client's strengths and weaknesses in either understanding or producing:
  - grammatical structures, i.e. morphology and syntax
  - word forms, i.e. phonology and phonetics.
- *Content* is the 'linguistic expression of what we have in mind' (Lahey 1988, p. 11). It is related to the understanding and producing of words that carry the required meaning:
  - vocabulary that is appropriate to objects, events and actions
  - the relationships of objects, events and actions.
- *Use* (or pragmatics) means the way in which language is used to interact with others. This involves the understanding and manipulation of the communication between individuals such as:
  - 'norms' of communication, e.g. turn-taking, use of gesture and facial expression, use of spatial and postural adjustments for different contexts
  - supralinguistic information carried by vocal tone and intonation patterns
  - conversational patterns, e.g. making statements, commands, requests, attending to the topic under discussion, saying appropriate things in response, knowing what kind of and how much information to offer, etc.
  - identifying and using inference (including humour) and problem-solving through language.

As well as spoken or signed language ability, you will need to investigate a child's or adult's literacy levels. The known links between slow phonological development and reading and writing problems (Stackhouse and Wells 1997), as well as the importance of understanding the possible loss of these skills after brain injury (Barry 1991), highlight the importance of this knowledge.

As well as exploring the language system directly, you will need to look carefully at those cognitive skills that are necessary for language to develop (Eysenck 2001). There is some controversy about how these skills link to language acquisition (Marschark et al. 1997), but it is clear that an understanding of the abilities of your clients in these areas will give you a better picture of the constraints under which their language systems have to function. So you will want to assess the following:

- Attention, which is the ability to focus on and remain focused on salient features of the situation in order for learning to take place (for a useful framework of levels of attention, see Cooper et al. 1978).
- Auditory and visual abilities: acuity, discrimination, memory.
- Short-term memory, which is the ability to retain information for long enough to allow it to make links and connections to other information stored in the brain.
- Conceptualization, which is learning the way in which the world can be grouped and categorized in order for it to make sense. An understanding of how things are the same and different, how they are organized into groups, how events are sequenced in time and how things are organized in space is vital for the growth of awareness and knowledge upon which language is built.
- Problem-solving: the ability to work out appropriate sequences of actions or events to arrive at a designated goal.
- Play: for appropriate play to develop, all the cognitive processes above are brought together. Through observation of a child's play you can gain an enormous amount of information about awareness, sociability, symbolic ability, conceptualization, problem-solving, etc. (see Jeffree 1996, for an outline of developmental sequences of play).

Finally, if dysphagia is one of the difficulties with which your client presents, you will need to ensure that you explore in detail (Royal College of Speech and Language Therapists or RCSLT 2003c):

- atypical patterns of sucking, eating, chewing, drinking, swallowing
- consistencies of food and liquid that are safe to swallow
- clinically significant signs related to problems of aspiration
- the progress of the bolus through the oral, pharyngeal and swallowing stages
- through a thorough understanding of bedside assessment and other assessment approaches using equipment such as videofluoroscopy or electromyography.

The information-gathering process may take place before, during or after you have seen the client. The chances are it will occur during all three periods and for quite a time after you have seen someone for the first session. As for all clinical processes, it is not finite – there are always new pieces of information to be discovered. It is impossible to learn everything about a person and his or her problem, but if you take a whole-person view and tap as many sources of information as possible, you will begin gradually to build up a picture of your client and his or her needs.

The initial contact

The word 'contact' rather than 'interview' has been used deliberately, because the latter presupposes a formal, fact-gathering process, which may not be the best way forward for the person with whom you are dealing. 'Contact' suggests a more open-ended coming together which may not be directly face to face, but could be observation from a distance, information gathering on the phone or informal, unstructured meetings, as well as the more commonly expected question-and-answer format.

The initial contact is where you are going to gather much, but not all, of the information that you have just considered. Before you meet your client for the first time you must consider your moral and ethical duty as a professional. The RCSLT (1996, p. 18) comments:

> Speech and language therapists should: respect the legal, social and moral norms of the society in which they work . . . refrain from discrimination on the basis of race, religion, gender or any other considerations . . . respect the needs and opinions of the clients to whom a duty of care is owed.

Consent to treatment

Before engaging with the client, you need to ensure that he or she is happy to undergo the process of assessment and possible therapy. This means that the person must understand, as far as possible, what you are going to do. The client needs to give *informed consent*, which suggests that the clinician has offered a range of treatment options and explained possible outcomes to the best of her knowledge (see RCSLT 1996, pp. 206–8, for further discussion).

It is also important that you think carefully about the concept of *confidentiality*:

> Speech and language therapists must maintain professional confidentiality with regard to their clients, and must refrain from disclosing information about a client which has been learned directly or indirectly in a professional capacity . . . where information is shared with professional colleagues or any other person it is the speech and language therapist's responsibility to ensure that such people appreciate that the information is being imparted in strict professional confidence.
>
> College of Speech and Language Therapists (1991, p. 18)

Some points to consider before you make the initial contact are:

• How will you make contact?
• In what context will the information be gathered?

- To whom will you speak?
- How much time will you have?
- What will be your aims and objectives for this contact?
- Based on these, what information will it be necessary to know?
- What will be your client's expectations and perceptions of the problem?

How will you make contact?

The way in which clients are contacted could be influenced by your work setting, your time and your own style of approach. If this is an inpatient contact, you might phone the ward to make arrangements to come and see the client. The ward staff will then be responsible for telling the client that you are coming. In an outpatient department or a community clinic there may be specific procedures, such as a standard letter or card, that the department you are working in sends to the prospective client. This may give some information about the appointment and what might be expected on arrival at the speech and language clinic. If the client has been seen before, you might choose to make contact by phone or a more personal letter. Remember that the way in which the client has been contacted can have an effect on his or her feelings about the meeting with you.

The context of the contact and to whom you will talk

There are many situations in which you may see the client and/or carer(s). Some of these are ideal, well-planned and well-prepared settings, others may be awkward and uncomfortable and the space, noise levels, availability of equipment and so on may be outside your control. Your client may be seen:

- in bed or in a side room on a hospital ward
- in a community or other 'clinical' space
- at home
- in a day-care setting
- in a school
- in a large and airy room
- in a small and dismal space
- on his or her own
- with one other person
- with the whole family
- in almost any other setting that you can think of.

Wherever the face-to-face contact is, you must be aware of the effect that this environment is likely to have on the comfort or discomfort of the people involved – including yourself. The nature of the information that you gather will also be influenced by the setting. In a very public space it would be inappropriate to talk about overly personal issues. Discussing language problems with your client or conducting tests where he or she may fail in some areas will need a quiet and confidential setting. A large room is necessary if a whole family is to be seen. The availability of toys and space is essential to encourage a child's play.

Aims and objectives (goals or outcomes)

You do not need to know your client in order to establish aims and objectives. The very limited information you may have on your referral letter will be enough to give you a starting point for writing a plan for your initial contact.

Your *aims* or general intentions will be to gather information and to form some opinion of what the particular issues are, from both the client's and the carers' viewpoints, as well as from your own. Breakwell (1990, p. 1) points out that an effective interaction 'helps you see what is happening from the other's point of view as well as your own. This helps you predict what might happen next'.

The areas that you hope to explore might be some or all of the following (after Priestley and McGuire 1983):

- The person: age, appearance, mobility, interests, attitudes, feelings, expectations, level of functioning, etc.
- The context: school, home, work, neighbourhood, culture, etc.
- The family: family members, family structure, support, relationships between family members, etc.
- The problem: is there a problem? Who is most concerned? Duration and course of the problem, help previously sought, others involved in problem, effects on life of those involved.

Objectives are specific *goals* of the meeting or hoped-for *outcomes* of the encounter. The word 'objectives' will be used, although, in different settings, you may find the words 'goals' or 'learning outcomes'. It is best to consider objectives from a specific point of view:

- From the point of view of the client: what will he or she have done during the session that will meet the aims?
- From the point of view of interested others: what have the parents done or asked to meet their concerns about schooling or family plans?
- From your point of view: what have you done or provided that will meet the aim of finding out about the problem?

You will also need to consider before you see the client what *procedures* you expect to undertake in order to meet your own aims and objectives, and what activities or *methods* will be used. All of these will be contained in your initial plan (Figure 3.5).

You have been asked to see John who is 2 years and 10 months old and who has been described by his doctor as being uncommunicative. You will be seeing John and his mother in your community clinic where you have the available space and equipment that is likely to be appropriate for a child of this age. You write the following aims and objectives.

Aims
1. To obtain information on John's development from his mother.
2. To assess John's level of play.
3. To identify John's method of communication – with his mother and with the clinician.
4. To get an impression of John's level of language comprehension.

Objectives
1. That John will have been at ease in this strange setting.
2. That John's mother will have given information about his development and felt able to express her concerns about him and his speech.
3. That John will have completed a test of his play abilities as well as played with a range of toys (a) with his mother, (b) on his own, and (c) with the clinician.
4. That John will have responded to direct requests for objects or actions from (a) his mother and (b) the clinician.

Procedures
1. Observe communication between John and his mother while they engage in play using general play equipment.
2. Note John's ability to continue playing when his mother is engaged in discussion.
3. Become involved in play with John and suggest sorting and matching.
4. Give John specific directions during play.
5. If appropriate, use more formal assessment approach.

Methods
1. Set out garage and cars, farm and farmhouse, building blocks and bag of well-known objects (have some pictures that match these objects available).
2. Use Symbolic Play Test to formally assess play skills if appropriate.
3. Use Derbyshire Language Scheme for comprehension probing – you may need to adapt questions to fit the game being played.
4. Use developmental chart for planning questions about John's development.
5. Seek permission to tape record and video record for data analysis.

Figure 3.5 Example of a plan for an initial contact.

Moving through the session

Openings

The first hurdle to cross is that of names – will you use first names or surnames? You must be sensitive to forms of address that are appropriate for the ages or cultural backgrounds of the people whom you are seeing.

Once you have managed to establish names, you may wish to put the person at ease by asking some general questions, e.g. about the journey, the manner of arrival, the weather, etc. This should be carefully timed and not too long (although you may find this a very useful way of making your first informal assessment of the client's speech and language abilities).

After the introductions, you should explain to the client and/or carers what you have planned for the session and what they may expect from this initial contact. Most people will come not knowing what to expect but having some hopes and fears of their own. Giving an outline of what will occur removes the anxiety of the unknown and begins the process of rapport building that is so vital for this and subsequent contacts.

Asking questions

It is important to understand the power of questions either to encourage free and in-depth discussion or to stop the flow of an interaction and reduce responses to their most minimal. Hargie et al. (1994) suggest that questioning is one of the most important skills in social interaction. The nature and functions of questions should be further explored through their book. The important thing to remember in this initial contact is that open and closed questions elicit different responses (Figure 3.6).

The clinician is talking to John's mother about his development and home situation.

Closed questions	**Response**
How old is John?	He's nearly 3
And has he got any brothers or sisters?	Yes, a sister
Oh, how old is his sister?	She's 18 months
And do they play together well?	Yes

Open questions	**Response**
Tell me some of the things John likes to do at home	Well he plays with his sister. They like to chase around the house now that she can walk
So how active is John?	Oh very active. And careless. He is always knocking his little sister over. I have to watch them all the time

---

Figure 3.6 Examples of open and closed questions.

Closed questions are less threatening to the client and to you because they give you control over the interaction. They are good for starting off the session, particularly if the client is a bit unsure, and they elicit useful factual information, such as age, address, medical condition, schooling, etc. *Open questions* give the client control over what to say. They allow the client to offer extended information, as well as thoughts and feelings about a situation. But this does mean that you have less control of where the questioning might lead. To use open questions competently requires a good degree of skill in reflecting, paraphrasing, clarifying and summarizing, which you will gain through courses and reading in the area of the development of counselling skills.

The skill in initial sessions is knowing when to move from one topic to another and how to lead the interaction so that the information that you are seeking is tapped. You will have some time restraints and you will need to feel that you know the client and his or her situation well enough to make a decision on where to go next. It could be that the client or carer is talking at length about an issue that concerns him or her. You may realize that this needs to be dealt with but that this initial session is possibly not the appropriate place to do so. How will you express this? How will you acknowledge the need to discuss it but at the same time encourage movement to other necessary topics? You may become aware that this is a problem that is outside your professional competence, so you will need to suggest that it is discussed elsewhere. How will you phrase this comment? This is where skills learned from books on counselling (e.g. Dalton 1994, Egan 1994, Street 1994) and in experiential workshops and courses can be used.

Closing the session

Closing the session involves:

- stopping the flow of what is happening
- summarizing what has been done
- inviting questions
- giving a clear indication of what will happen next
- leaving the client/carers feeling that you have given them quality time.

What must be avoided is abrupt, 'run-out-of-time' endings with clients bustled out through the door, not knowing what they have accomplished and what will now happen.

Endings are difficult times for inexperienced clinicians. The pressure of having to say what will happen next is great and many clients may expect instant answers to their problems. The importance of setting the scene at the opening of the session now becomes clear. If you have carefully explained that you will gather information and make informal assessments of what the problems are, and involve the client and carer in what will happen next, it will be easier to share your findings with them and negotiate possibilities for future action. Your options are to offer:

- further assessment
- some ongoing intervention, with the client, the carer or both, or via a programme planned with the school or other professionals

- a self-help programme for which the client and/or carer is fully responsible
- a review after a period of time in which further information can be gathered or development can take place
- a referral on to another, more appropriate, professional
- support via a self-help group
- no further contact.

Any of these may be acceptable to clients if they are explored with them and any other relevant people, and if adequate and careful explanations are given for the decision.

The initial contact is now over. You will realize that this first meeting will have been crucial in the formation of a relationship with this client and his or her family or carers. The client will also have been forming an opinion of you while you have been making your assessment of his or her language.

You may be feeling that this session did not go as well as planned. Certain areas of difficulty may not have been assessed, questions may not have been asked, the words used to express some ideas may have been inappropriate. You may be left feeling that you still do not really understand what the problem is. Reflection and evaluation of this nature are vital skills that will encourage your development as a clinician. If you do not evaluate what you have done, what was adequate and what not, you will be unable to plan adequately for future meetings. Remember that self-awareness is often painful. If you are objective in the process of self-evaluation, just as you are expected to be as a speech and language clinician, you can use the reflection process as a learning tool. A framework for self-evaluation such as the one below will help you to maintain a professional distance:

- How do I feel? Do I feel comfortable, anxious, depressed, exhilarated? Why? What am I basing these feelings on?
- What did I do well? How useful was my plan, did I open well, ask questions well, explore relevant areas, allow the client time, use techniques appropriately, enable the client to make choices and be fully involved, etc.?
- How well can I evaluate the outcomes of the session? Did I have appropriate goals and criteria for success, did I record well enough to identify how the client succeeded?
- What would I have liked to do differently? What were the weaknesses in my planning, my running of the session, my ability to relate to the client, my ability to enable the client to succeed?
- How could I have changed?
- What additional knowledge and skills do I need in order to make these changes?

There will be ongoing meetings with many clients and, as with any relationship, trust and understanding will develop over time. As has already been stressed, assessment is a continuing process, so any information you feel that you have missed can be collected later, and new, previously unconsidered information will emerge. The process of assessment is challenging, but it is also one of the most interesting and stimulating activities in the speech and language therapy profession.

Data collection

What do we mean by the word 'data'?

Data are a group of known or ascertained facts from which conclusions are drawn and on which discussions are based. During the initial meeting and all subsequent sessions, you will be interested in gathering and recording data related to the behaviour of your clients and others. Data collection is more complex than you might think and it is important to understand the possibilities and pitfalls of this task. (See Miller 1981, Lahey 1988, Ingram 1989, Crystal and Varley 1998, among others, for useful discussion of data collection.)

Clinical bias

Remember as you start to gather your data that you may be unwittingly biasing the collection process by:

- your own age, sex and race
- your personality, e.g. anxiety, authoritarianism, etc.
- conducting the session at a particular time of day, in a particular setting, etc.
- unknowingly modelling the behaviours you expect from your client
- having an expectation of certain outcomes from your client and consequently asking questions that will bias the answer, e.g. 'Do you read to your child?', where the expectation is that the parent should do so and he or she will give the answer 'Yes' to please you.

In some instances you can do very little to alter the possible biases, e.g. if a client decides not to tell you certain things because they think you are too young. However, you can be careful about timing the data collection, managing your own anxiety, asking questions objectively, etc.

Initial considerations

You need to consider:

- what behaviours you wish to investigate
- where you wish to investigate them
- how you will investigate them
- how you will record your information.

What to investigate

We have already covered the general areas and sources of information in our consideration of what to assess. When you are with a client, you will probably want to take special note of those aspects of behaviour that contribute to the possible speech and language disorder. So you may be gathering data on:

- communication:
  - interaction
  - communicative intent
  - non-verbal skills
- speech:
  - phonetic inventory
  - articulation
  - phonological system
- language:
  - syntax
  - morphology
  - phonological processing
  - pragmatic use of language
- cognition:
  - object recognition
  - perception
  - attention and listening
  - memory
  - reasoning
- swallowing:
  - motor control of articulators
  - chewing
  - swallowing
  - choking
  - aspiration.

Where to investigate

The environment plays an important part in influencing people's behaviour. Any setting that makes the client feel uncomfortable will alter the amount or type of that behaviour. A child who is relaxed and playing happily in a known and comfortable space is more likely to be talkative and spontaneous than one in a new and unknown room. Visual or auditory distractions can create a less than ideal environment for the collection of speech data.

Influences on the context

The purpose of your data collection and the nature of the data to be collected may influence the context, e.g. if you wish to use instrumentation such as a laryngograph, the client will have to come to the equipment. This may be an alien environment and you will need to work extra hard to help your client feel as comfortable as possible. If you are doing a screening assessment, the nursery setting might be the ideal place to watch a child interacting and playing and note down a few examples of his or her spontaneous speech, as well as noticing what he or she seems to understand of the language used. If, however, you need to decide the level of this child's comprehension or the nature of his or her phonological difficulty, you will have to structure the setting and the input in order to assess the specified area.

How to investigate

The way in which you gather data will vary depending on whether you are doing a formal or informal assessment. Many formal assessment procedures will provide you with information on how to gather and analyse data. So in this section we focus on more informal, observational procedures. We believe that you will need to gather information informally as a basis for making hypotheses about the nature of the problem, and you might then use the more formal tests to follow up on these initial possibilities. You will need to understand your client's strengths and weaknesses in both language comprehension and expression. Look out for books that give ideas on assessing particular areas of the linguistic system, such as that by McDaniel et al. (1996) on assessing children's syntax or Harley's (1995) book on the psychology of language, which has an excellent chapter on comprehension. Books that help you understand what you need to assess, such as that by Bishop (1997) on understanding and by Black and Chiat (2003) on rules of language, are essential reading to enable you to plan your assessment.

Expressive language

What constitutes a representative language sample?

Length

The sample must be long enough to give a picture of the type of words a client uses, the way in which he or she structures sentences and the way in which words are pronounced. As people may produce words differently on different occasions, and may limit their topics to those that they feel competent to manage, the larger the sample the better. But time is a factor that prevents you from obtaining ideal data, so you may adopt a more realistic target of around 200 utterances or about 30 minutes of conversation (Miller 1981, Crystal et al. 1989). At times, it may be appropriate to have a sample of single-word utterances, which may be collected in a phonological or articulatory assessment. It is also important to have a sample of connected speech where you can observe the way in which particular combinations of words affect the client's ability to sequence and articulate the sounds of speech. Connected speech samples are essential to make some analysis of your client's grammatical abilities.

As well as obtaining a sample of the form of your client's utterances, it is necessary to have data that can allow for the analysis of some of the pragmatic aspects of language. You will therefore need to record both the client and yourself or another conversational partner to analyse features of the discourse.

Elicited vs spontaneous

Different samples will be gathered from these two approaches, so it is best to consider using both. To elicit a language sample you might use a formal test such as the Action Picture Test (Renfrew 2001). Remember that elicited language can be unrepresentative, lead to single-word utterances and fail to capture words that the client uses regularly. Spontaneous samples can be difficult to gather and can be limited in the number or type of utterances. Conversely, spontaneous samples can give a good indication of the child's or adult's ability in connected utterances, whereas elicited samples can focus on those aspects of language that are less likely to occur in a fairly short spontaneous sample.

Ways of encouraging speech

Eliciting

- Demand: 'What's this?'
- Encourage: 'Oh, here is a . . . .'
- Sentence completion: 'The girl is eating the . . . .'
- Imitation: 'This is an apple. It's an . . . ?'
- Model offered: 'This is a girl, this is an apple. The girl is eating the . . . ?'
- Forced alternative: 'Is it an apple or a carrot?'
- Recall: 'Now you tell me about it'.

Conversation

A general conversation is an ideal way of obtaining data that are naturalistic and it can also be manipulated by the nature of the questions that you ask. When engaged in conversation with your client, remember the following:

- Listen
- Be patient – don't overpower with requests, questions, etc.
- Follow the client's lead
- Value the client – pay full attention to what he or she does or says
- Do not play the fool, i.e. do not ask questions to which you obviously know the answer
- Consider the client's perspective.

Play (after Miller 1981)

* Say nothing
* Play in parallel
* Interact during play with little speech
* Interact during play with speech.

Collecting data on language comprehension

Bishop (1997) has provided a framework for analysing comprehension, which involves considering each stage in the process of transforming a set of speech sounds into a meaningful message. Using this framework as the basis for generating questions about how and why a client is hearing, identifying, analysing and making sense of the incoming information will enable you to make 'educated' hypotheses about comprehension while you gather your information by the following means:

* General observation, which will involve, for example, watching the child when in the nursery: how quickly does he or she respond to directions? How much does he or she need to observe the other children? Or watching the adult with learning difficulties with a member of the care staff: how many times is the direction repeated? How much physical prompting is the staff member using? etc.
* General conversation where the client's ability to follow the social language of conversation and to respond appropriately (maybe through nodding or gesture) to comments and queries such as 'How are you feeling today?' or 'It's lovely and warm outside, isn't it?' will give valuable information.
* Yes/no responses where the client's ability to understand when information is correct or incorrect and whether a positive or negative response is needed can be identified, such as 'Is that tea you've got?' (when it is coffee) or 'Is your name Tom?' (when it is Peter). Remember that, for some clients, the problem may lie in their inability to generate the correct verbal or gestural response to the question, i.e. an expressive problem, rather than a lack of understanding of the question. For many of these people, their obvious awareness via facial expression, gesture, etc. will show that they know they have given an incorrect response. But, again, there will be those who cannot convey this to you.
* Word–picture/object matching, which can be done in play or in general conversation, e.g. 'Shall I give you your *glasses*?', 'Do you want to play with *teddy*?', while watching where the client looks, or more formally 'Where is the cup?', 'Where is the pen?', etc. This can be built up from single words to more complex and longer sentences; see tests for adults and children such as Western Aphasia Battery (Keresz 1982) or the Derbyshire Language Scheme (Knowles and Masidlover 1982). Remember that, for some clients, comprehension will be more difficult in isolated speech than in more natural conversational settings.

- Giving directions such as 'show me your arm', 'put the ball in the box', 'point to the object on the right of the spoon', etc. can be used to probe language comprehension. You must be careful to build up slowly to the more complex commands which might use concepts that are not understood (e.g. right vs left) or are linguistically difficult, such as embedded phrases like 'show me the man in the red hat who is walking down the road'. See comprehension tests such as the Test for Reception of Grammar (TROG – Bishop 1989) for examples of increasingly difficult syntactic constructions.
- Asking questions such as 'what?, who?, where?, how?', which require the client to work out what is being requested through an understanding of the question form. For many clients these question forms require more linguistic processing than they can manage given their language problem.
- Checking understanding of inference by asking questions that go beyond the literal meaning apparent in the context. Questions such as 'Is Uncle Chris a man or a woman?' require the ability to attach gender to certain words. 'Was Jane late for work?', following a story where it was previously mentioned that the time was already 9.15 and Jane's boss would be furious with her, demands the ability to relate new to previous information. 'Arthur walked to the shops where he met his brother and they talked about his wife' can present an enormous amount of difficulty to a client who cannot sort out which pronoun relates to whom. Harley (1995, p. 216) comments that 'one of the main tools of comprehension is to sort out to what pronouns refer'.
- Identifying knowledge of intended meanings. Some children or adults will have difficulty using additional factors such as the situation, facial expression, tone of voice, as a way of obtaining underlying meaning and will take the literal representation of the sentence as 'fact'. You can check whether this is the case by giving a verbal message with an 'alternative' facial expression 'Oh dear, I've broken my favourite plate' with a smile. 'Do you think I am worried about that?' A formal test using this approach is Understanding Ambiguity by Rinaldi (1996).

Remember that comprehension requires intact attention, listening skills and memory, and your client's inability to respond appropriately might well be as a result of a problem in one of these areas. Children or adults who lack a great deal of experience will have little world knowledge to help them work out what is being said. Their comprehension of language will thus be limited. Bilingual children whose background experience may be very different from that of their school peers may need a lot of help in developing their understanding of some English words. As a speech and language clinician, it is very important in your assessment of a client's comprehension that you take into account all these factors and systematically explore all the possible reasons why he or she is having difficulties in understanding language.

Recording of data

When you collect a sample of language for analysis, it is vital that you record. You may do this by writing down what you hear or see during the contact with the client or you may use video or audio recording, depending on what is available. You may fill in a pre-prepared checklist or a chart of some kind as you proceed through the session. Whatever you do, it is important that you: (1) prepare for the recording beforehand; (2) record systematically; and (3) have recording equipment that is of good quality. Remember that attentive listening and observation skills can pick up more information than the most sophisticated of recording devices. You can watch accompanying non-verbal behaviour, gain information on production via lip shapes or muscle tension, and note interactive exchanges that are too subtle for a video to detect. Your data may lend itself to either qualitative or quantitative analysis, and it is best to think beforehand about which of these might be the more appropriate. *Quantitative* data, such as timing of utterances, counting of dysfluencies, recording of pitch variations, etc., can be used to compare clients with either normative data or their own previous performances. *Qualitative* data are necessary to give a picture of the nature of the communicative strengths and weaknesses. Each has its place and, for a full assessment, both should be used.

Transcription

Once the information has been gathered you are ready to produce a transcript as a precursor to analysis of your data. To transcribe is to write out and arrange information in full. Your transcription may be:

- orthographic, i.e. recorded in the accepted script of the language
- phonetic, i.e. using standard symbols such as those of the International Phonetic Alphabet (Ladefoged 2001) to identify the nature of the sounds spoken
- broad or narrow phonetic script, i.e. either a transcription that has little detail (broad), or that which shows phonetic detail (such as aspiration, length, airstream mechanism, etc.) through the use of a wide variety of symbols and diacritics.

Orthographic transcriptions are used when the analysis is to be grammatical or conversational, whereas phonetic script is commonly used to identify speech characteristics. The transcript may consist of just the language gathered or the accompanying situational or behavioural information can also be recorded.

Perkins and Howard (1995) cited Kelly and Local (1989, p. 26) who say that 'at the beginning of work on language material we can't . . . know beforehand what is going to be important'. It is always amazing that patterns that have been entirely missed during the process of face-to-face discussion and elicitation can emerge from a transcription.

A good transcription allows for evaluation of change over time. The effort spent at this point in making a good transcription is therefore important in decisions about where to go next and in identifying change. Transcriptions must be objective, recording what is heard and seen, and avoiding the possibility of bias. However, you are using your own listening and observation skills as well as your ability in applying the forms of transcription, such as phonetic script, and consequently the transcript is unlikely to be as objectively reliable as you would wish. The best way to overcome this bias is to have the data analysed by more than one person. Information that can be said to be reliable is that which is agreed by at least two, if not more, observers.

There are numerous texts that give information on how to proceed in transcription, and these should be consulted to help you produce the most valid data for analysis (see Crystal 1982, Grunwell 1987, Kelly and Local 1989). To a certain extent transcription will be directed by your general hypotheses about the problem. Whether the speech sample will be transcribed in orthographic script, broad phonetic script or narrow phonetic script will depend on whether a semantic/grammatical, phonological or articulatory investigation is being conducted. But you must always remember that these subsystems of language are closely connected and that a disorder in, for example, the use of syntax may be evidence of a reduced phonological ability being masked by the child choosing to use simple language forms. Remember also that a decision to use a particular form of data, e.g. single words, can bias the analysis unless it is supported by other data, e.g. connected speech. Crystal (1982) gives an outline of the main features needed in a transcription (Table 3.3):

1. Each sentence used by the client and by the clinician is placed on a separate line and preferably numbered.
2. A wide margin is left on the right-hand side of the page in order to comment on additional necessary information, e.g. the visual referent for the language, the gestures being used alongside or instead of speech, etc.
3. Prosodic features are identified (marking of tone units, the direction of the nuclear tone, other prominent stressed syllables and degrees of pause length) in order to understand the way in which grammar is being organized.

Table 3.3 Example of an orthographic transcription

Example:			
1	T	is that a 'red car/	Points to the green car
2	C	no 'nòt/	Shakes his head
3	T	teddy thought it was 'red/	Jumps teddy up and down
4	C	silly teddy/	
		'green/	Holds car in front of teddy

Reliability in transcription

The less intelligible the speech of your client, the more difficult it is to be sure that you have correctly transcribed the speech data. The only way to be sure that the phonetic transcription is accurate is by consensus – others must also transcribe aspects of the data (Shriberg and Lof 1991). Remember that no one can get narrow phonetic transcription 'right', so there is no shame in your seeking help from others. Obviously, the most useful help could come from a clinical linguist, but other speech and language clinicians or students can help to establish the presence or absence of certain features in the speech of your client. Does this mean that if you are on your own you should not bother to make a phonetic transcription? No. Perkins and Howard (1995, p. 31) explain that 'the very act of transcription, regardless of how accurately one transcribes, makes the transcriber pay very close attention to the speech and language data, thus usually prompting a number of testable hypotheses about the client's abnormal communication behaviour'.

Non-verbal transcriptions

So far we have assumed that your client has some verbal behaviour to transcribe. But many clients whom you may see will be non-verbal. What are you to do about them? This is where video recordings can be of such benefit. Within an interaction there are numerous behaviours to be recorded on paper: eye contact, facial expression, gesture, vocalization, posture – all give indications of the communicative ability of your clients. (For an excellent example of such a transcription, see Wootton 1989.)

Instrumental measurement techniques

Instrumental methods are used to provide objective data on a number of acoustic, aerodynamic and physiological features of speech (Wood and Hardcastle 2000).

   Table 3.4 gives an outline of some of the instruments that may be available to you, what they measure and when you might use them.

Data analysis and evaluation

What is analysis?

Analysis is the systematic examination of the information that you have gathered and determination of the general nature of the behaviours that you see.

   Before proceeding to consider ways in which you might systematically examine the data that you have gathered, you must first be alert to the possibility of bias. We have commented on bias before, but it is important enough to revisit in the light of the process of analysis that you are about to undertake. So remember you must set out to minimize bias by:

Table 3.4 Instrumental measurement in speech and language disorders

Instrument	What measured	Why used
Electropalatograph	Lingual–palatal contact patterns	Visual feedback for articulatory placements
Endoscope	Glottal aperture	Vocal fold movement
Nasometer	Nasal-oral airflow	Velopharyngeal competence
Videofluoroscope	Radiograph of supralaryngeal cavities	Swallowing difficulties, velopharyngeal incompetence
Videostroboscope	Viewing vocal fold behaviour in real time	Detection of possible cause of voice disorder
Spectrograph	Duration, formant frequencies	Identification of phonetic features of speech production
Visi-Speech, Speech Viewer, etc.	Edits real speech and synthesizes artificial speech	Gives visual feedback on parameters of speech production

- being aware that you are subject to it
- using and keeping taped or videoed information
- sharing findings with a colleague
- standardizing your own behaviour during assessment as much as possible to avoid giving additional cues to your clients.

To make your data more manageable, to find what you are looking for more easily and to begin the process of understanding the nature of what you are seeing, it is wise to organize what you have recorded in a systematic way.

Procedures for organizing data

Linear arrangement

Alphabetical ordering

This is of use when you have a number of single words that you need to be able to find easily. It may also give you clues about the variability or stability of production of a particular initial phoneme. A set of phonological data or single words uttered by a child in the early stages of expressive language development can initially be arranged in this way (Table 3.5).

Chronological ordering

For longitudinal data, e.g. utterances collected by a parent at home over months, play behaviour seen at nursery over a number of weeks, or changes

Table 3.5 Examples of alphabetical ordering of data

Word spoken	Child's pronunciation
Adam	'de
apple	?epu
baby	bebe
bottle	bobo
bread	be

in extent or range of movement over time in a client with Parkinson's disease, it is important and useful to present the information in a clearly dated chronology, e.g.:

Child with developmental delay

2.2.93	Picked up ball and dropped it five times.
4.4.93	Transferred ball from one hand to the other once.
24.6.93	Holds objects in either hand and transfers from one to the other easily.

Categorical arrangement

To gain information about the nature of the behaviours that you have observed, you may wish to organize them in particular categories, e.g. word classes for semantic or grammatical information, semantic fields, types of play, etc. (Table 3.6).

Table 3.6 Examples of simple categorical arrangement of data

1. Organizing words understood by a child into semantic fields (e.g. people)

Family	Others	Jobs	Character
Mummy	Friend	Milkman	Happy
Daddy	Man	Postman	Nasty
John			

2. Organizing words used by a child into word classes

Nouns	Verbs	Adjectives
Baby	Go	Hot
Boy	Give	Nice
Biscuit	Yumyum (eat)	
Car		
Dog		

More complex organizations of language behaviour will be needed to identify grammatical categories or phonological processes and you are strongly advised to become competent at these. Books such as those by Black and Chiat (2003), Crystal et al. (1989), Fabb (1994) and Grunwell (1985) are highly recommended (Figure 3.7).

(a)

the	man	in	a	hat	is	playing	on	the	new	violin
D	N		D	N	Aux	V	Pr	D	A	N

| NP | | Pr | | NP | | | | | | |

NP, S   V   PP, A

(b)

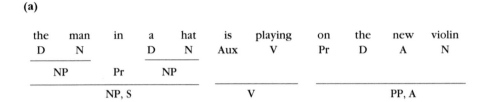

(c)

1. Syllable structure process: final consonant deletion		**2. Substitution process: stopping of fricatives**	
Target	Child's realization	Target	Child's realization
/kat/	[ka]	/sun/	[tu]
/pig/	[pi]	/farm/	[ka]
/haus/	[hau]	/shoe/	[tu]
/bath/	[ba]		

Figure 3.7 Examples of grammatical and phonological arrangements of data: (a) following the LARSP (Crystal et al., 1989); (b) in the form of a tree diagram (Fabb, 1994); (c) two phonological processes found to be operating in a child with learning difficulties (Grunwell, 1985).

Always remember when you are analysing grammatical constructions that characteristics of spoken English may follow an unusual form, not because the client is disordered, but because he or she has another language as the mother tongue. Word order may be affected. In Bengali, for example, the basic subject–verb–object structure that we are so used to is replaced by a subject–object–verb structure, or words such as negatives will appear at the end of the sentence (see Duncan 1989, for further examples).

Coding

This is simply a way of identifying when particular behaviours occur within a continuous sample, e.g. when noting the occurrence of an initiation or a response within a conversation, one may simply mark an I or an R by the noticed behaviour. Or, in identifying the number of repetitions or prolongations that are occurring, one may mark an R or a P at the point of occurrence. These can then be counted to arrive at a quantity of the particular behaviour and this can be compared with what may be expected, or to some criterion previously identified (Figure 3.8).

(a)

	Speaker	Utterance	Coding
1	Therapist	/what have you been 'doing today/	I
2	Paul	/I went 'out/	R
3	Therapist	/where did you 'go/	I
4	Paul	/'swimming/ /yeh 'swimming/	R

(long pause during which therapist waits to see if Paul will add more information)

	Speaker	Utterance	Coding
5	Therapist	/would you like to 'tell me something about the swimming/	I
6	Paul	/'no/	R

(b)

```
            R          P          P          R
    P     I I I I thinkI  w:::::ill go to the c::::::::in  e e e ema
```

Figure 3.8 Examples of coding language behaviours: (a) lack of initiations in the conversation of a brain-injured young adult; (b) identifying repetitions and prolongations in stuttered speech.

Profiling

> A profile is a chart containing an organized collection of categories, which represent the structural contrasts available in a language – the various sounds, grammatical patterns, lexical items and so on.
>
> Crystal (1982, p. 5)

The following are some examples of well-known profiles in speech and language assessment:

- Language Assessment, Remediation and Screening Procedure (LARSP – Crystal et al. 1989), which is presented in a single-page profile chart that contains information from the grammatical analysis of the data. Crystal stipulates that a profile should:
  - provide a comprehensive description of the client's data
  - provide an organized grading of the data
  - show the influences that operate on the client's language as he or she interacts with the interlocutor (Crystal 1982).
- Vocal Profile Analysis Scheme (VPAS), which was developed from work by Laver in 1968 (Wirz and Beck 1995) and provides a framework for analysis of both normal and disordered voice.
- The psycholinguistic profile (Stackhouse and Wells 1997), which provides a way of considering how the speech and language problems may arise from possible breakdowns or lack of development in language input, storage or output. Psycholinguistic processing models such as those of Levelt (1989) enable you to visualize what might be happening when language is being decoded or encoded by the brain.

It must be remembered, however, that a profile is purely a chart and that anyone can devise a chart to provide an appropriate examination of the data that are available. Dodd (1995), for example, provides a profile to pull together a number of different aspects of the linguistic system for contrast and comparison of information. She offers a diagnostic chart that looks at articulation of phones, phonological processes and rules, severity, and causal or maintenance factors. We use an approach similar to this later in the chapter as a way of comparing information from two clients.

The ability to collect and organize information in the above ways presupposes knowledge and ability in identification and description of behaviour gained through the study of linguistics, psychology, medical sciences, etc. There is no shortcut to these abilities. Study and careful training of your own visual and auditory perceptual processes is the only way to achieve the necessary degree of accuracy in assessment.

Evaluation of information

You now have in front of you a good sample of data related to the problem that your client has brought to you. You have collected and organized the data in an appropriate form so that they can be clearly seen and considered. What will you now do with the data? You need to evaluate what you have in front of you. What is the meaning of what you see and how can you arrive at useful conclusions from the information you have? Think of a jigsaw analogy – you have collected most, if not all, of the pieces, and now you are beginning to put them together in the hope that you will be able to make sense of the picture that they are forming. There are several ways of doing this.

Counting

A useful starting point is through the simple practice of counting. Counting how many times a particular behaviour occurs can be useful information in terms of the strength of that behaviour. A child who uses 20 nouns in the course of a 15-minute interaction will be different from one who uses 10 nouns, 7 verbs and 3 adjectives, although the word count is the same. Both of these children will be very different from the child who uses only three words in the same time and this child will differ from one who uses 3 words but 17 communicative gestures. A profile such as LARSP uses a simple count as the way to identify how much of the sample follows a particular theme or pattern. Thus, you can note how often the child uses a SVC (subject-verb–complement) structure versus how often he uses a SVCA (subject-verb–complement–adverbial) as a means of assessing how complex his utterances are.

Communicative competence

The second and a most useful approach to evaluation of the data is to look for what the client can do well – how well can he get his message across. So, for example, an analysis of the pragmatic functions of the conversation of a client with aphasia may well show that this person is questioning, requesting, stating, negating, etc., despite few full grammatical utterances (Table 3.7). You might also notice this client's competence in repair, turn-taking or maintaining a topic. Or you may be analysing information from a video of a mother interacting with her non-verbal child. Here you see that the child and mother are sharing attention to objects and events in the environment and this allows the parent to identify what the child needs. Some useful tools for identifying pragmatic features in adults or children with language disorders are the Conversation Analysis Profile for People with Aphasia (CAPPA – Whitworth et al. 1997) and the Test of Pragmatic Language (Phelps-Terasaki and Phelps-Gunn 1992).

Error analysis

Just counting the number of errors that a client produces is not particularly useful. However, an analysis of what the errors are and how they differ from

Table 3.7 Communicative competence in a conversational exchange

T	How are you today Mr B?	
B	Yes, yes OK/	Appropriate response
	You?/	Socially appropriate question – follows
	social rules	
T	I'm fine thanks. Tell me about your week	
B	Monday ... Tuesday ... out ... good/	Gives information
	Um ... ted ... um ... next one... no er Wezday	Self-repair
	No....not good/	Uses negation
T	Oh, were you ill on Wednesday?	
B	Say again/	Asks for repair
T	Ill ... poorly	
B	Ah, yes ... um (points to head)/	Continues conversation, adds information
T	But you're fine now?	
B	Yes ... thanks/	
	You ... picture?/	Initiates new topic

So, despite grammatical difficulties, this client B is competent in a conversational exchange

the expected behaviour is very useful in planning of treatment. It is also important to consider what the error is telling you. You can gather a great deal of information about the strategies that a client is using to overcome or circumvent a difficulty. Thus, in a phonological analysis, by noting that a child is fronting velar plosives (/k/ /g/ – [t] [d]) you have a notion of a possible systematic process being used by this child. You can now go on to see whether other groups of sounds are fronted, whether fronting takes place only in certain consonant–vowel relationships, etc. An adult with learning difficulties may be unable to complete the section on the TROG that deals with passives. You may notice an obvious understanding of the concept of actor and agent and an inability to give the actor role to an inanimate object. Thus 'the man is being pushed by the car' will be perceived as 'the man is pushing the car'. Such careful consideration of the direction of errors in speech and language will form the basis of your therapy. However, you must beware of over-simplification, e.g. you might listen to speech samples and 'phonemicize', i.e. 'tidy up', a client's phonetic output so that it fits into your prearranged programme of therapy (Gardner 1997). A narrow phonetic transcription of the speech of a client with complex difficulties may lead you to a realization that meaningful contrasts are being made in the speech system but by the use of non-English sounds (e.g. implosives, clicks, etc.) (Parker and Irlam 1995).

The example in Table 3.8 shows how you can use an error analysis with a child with semantic–pragmatic difficulties to identify an awareness of the nature of the topic, even though the ability to use the correct form of language to indicate cohesion is lacking. Cohesion is the tendency for communicative partners to relate their utterances to the topic under discussion and to relate back to what has been said beforehand. A child or adult with a conversational disability will find this difficult.

Table 3.8 Example of a careful analysis of errors in a language sample

1 Teacher	/Did you go 'out todày/	
2 Child	/Go òut/	Shows attending behaviour
3	/Go 'swìmming/	links to reason for often leaving the school building
4 Teacher	'no/	
5	You go swimming on tuèsday/	
6 Child	it my bìrthday/	Following previous train of thought as had a swimming party on her birthday

So, it becomes apparent that the child is actually attempting to participate in conversation even though these attempts appear to include errors of cohesion.

Overall analysis of strengths and areas of difficulty

If you have done some or all of the procedures above, you will have a knowledge of how often certain behaviours occur, how close to or far away from expected behaviours these are and how useful behaviours are in enabling the individual to communicate. You can begin to list the strengths and problems of this person's linguistic system as a preliminary to understanding what the important factors in the equation are that will eventually lead to decisions and priorities in management.

Case discussion: Mrs B

Mrs B was referred by her GP. She had had a stroke 9 months previously, had had some therapy in the early stages but had then been discharged. Her GP felt that she had shown some positive changes recently and that both she and her husband might benefit from therapy. You arranged to see Mrs B in the outpatient department of the local hospital. She was brought in by hospital transport, which meant that she had been collected very early from home and had been driven around for some time before you saw her. You therefore had only a short period of time with her and you formed some opinion about her difficulties.

Following this, you arranged to see Mrs B at home with her husband. In this setting, things were very different. Mrs B was much more relaxed and not tired. Her profile of strengths and areas of difficulty was now very different (Table 3.9).

Looking at Mrs B's profile so far, you are able to see that there has been much improvement in her comprehension, based on the information in her notes from 6 months previously. It is obvious that when she is tired, as she was when she came to clinic, she is unable to concentrate sufficiently and so cannot respond as well as when she is relaxed and alert. However, she still has some problems controlling her attention. It appears that her speech is very limited, but she shows some positive abilities in gesture. You feel you have started building a picture of her abilities, which you will need to extend before you can decide whether intervention is appropriate.

Table 3.9 Mrs B's strengths and weakesses in two different settings

(a) In the clinic

Strengths	Weaknesses
Showed willingness to communicate	Tired very easily and lost attention
Participated in social conversation by smiling and nodding appropriately	Unable to follow specific directions to point to certain objects
Used spontaneous gesture to indicate place (pointing) and tiredness (closed and opened eyes)	Very limited verbal output – some jargon words only. Unable to complete any formal assessment

(b) In the home

Strengths	Weaknesses
Gave many socially appropriate responses to questions using yes and no and some social phrases	Rather distracted by noises and activity in the home
Named familiar items with some groping, but intelligible	Tended to try to speak rather than use gesture
Interacted well with husband who was very supportive	Some tendency for husband to take control

Collating all information gathered

Once you have a wide range of information gathered from various sources and from your own assessments, you need a way to pull it all together so that you can begin to see what is and what is not important.

A grid similar to that used by Rustin et al. (1995) is one of a number of ways that can help you visualize the trends that are emerging from your data collection. What is important is to organize the information in such a way as to make your evaluative judgements and decisions follow logically from the data to which you have access.

Case discussion: Mrs B (continued)

Following further exploration of Mrs B's difficulties through informal and formal assessment, discussion with her and with Mr B and from some liaison with the speech and language clinician who had previously seen her and with her GP, you arrive at the overall picture shown in Figure 3.9.

It is possible to see from this grid that Mrs B's problems are primarily those of an environmental and social nature. True, she has major expressive language difficulties, but she is able to communicate her needs well. However, there are environmental changes that would enhance her ability and wish to communicate, such as reduction in background noise (the television) and increased independence. Encouragement in the use of her strengths – her gesture and writing – could compensate for some of her verbal difficulties. You are now clearer as to the direction that intervention may take. This overall visual picture has helped you to make sense of all the data that you have so far gathered.

Medical and developmental factors	Social/emotional factors
Has bronchitis often in winter	Mrs B gets upset if she is unable to
No extension of original stroke	achieve a task (as in the tests)
Mobility poor and no change over time	Mrs B very dependent on Mr B
Some reduction in hearing since stroke	Very social and socially capable, but
	goes out very little
Environmental factors	**Communication and language**
Home has been adapted but she finds	Good functional communication
it difficult to get out of the house	Comprehension good until long,
Husband is retired and has taken over	complex directions given
all household tasks	Hearing loss makes for difficulties when
No children and limited circle of friends	there is background noise
Previously Mrs B very keen on knitting	Limited verbal ability – only a few social
but now cannot manage	words intelligible – but Mrs B can
Television often on	spontaneously write single words when
	encouraged

Figure 3.9 Overall summary of Mrs B's difficulties.

Hypothesis generation and testing

A hypothesis is a clear statement about the relationship between two things (ideas, events, symptoms, etc.). Generating a statement of this sort helps you think about what you do and do not know about how these two factors relate and so will guide you to consider what further investigations may be necessary. The statement should be in some way testable, i.e. you should be able to think of a way to find out whether X really does relate to Y. Hypotheses should be made at all stages of assessment and intervention. By proceeding in this way you are deciding which pieces of jigsaw fit and which need to be discarded as you go along. It is easiest to see what is meant by a hypothesis by working through an example and showing what sort of hypotheses might be made at different stages of your assessment.

Case discussion: Lisa

Lisa is 7 years old. She was referred by her school, as she was having difficulty reading. The teacher said she had a slight speech problem but nothing they were worried about.

You have found that Lisa was known to the speech and language therapy service when she was between 3 and 4 years old. She presented with a fairly severe phonological delay, but this had remediated with therapy. At the time of her discharge she had a full phonetic inventory and the only phonological immaturities were some cluster reduction in /s/ clusters and gliding of /r/. There were no medical or developmental factors that were significant.

Hypothesis 1
The known relationship between phonological delay and reading difficulties suggests to you that this might be the area to investigate in detail when you see Lisa. You hypothesize that Lisa will show some metaphonological difficulties, i.e. she may have difficulties understanding that words are composed of syllables and that syllables are composed of parts such as the onset (the beginning consonant) and the rhyme (the following vowel and consonants).

Hypothesis 2
However, you have no information on the rest of her language system or on her general learning ability, so these could also play a role in her reading problem. You hypothesize that Lisa will show some delay in comprehension and/or expression of grammatical or semantic aspects of her language.

Hypothesis 3
As early reading ability may be linked to exposure to books, you hypothesize that Lisa's home has few books available or that Lisa had a past history of attention difficulties and/or reduced hearing or listening ability.

The initial contact with Lisa and her mother takes place in a clinical setting and you have assembled the appropriate materials: formal tests of metaphonology (rhyming, sound and syllable awareness using the Phonological Awareness Procedure - Gorrie and Parkinson 1995), comprehension of grammar (TROG - Bishop 1989) and vocabulary (British Picture Vocabulary Scale II - Dunn et al. 1997), as well as a range of dolls, books, paper and crayons, etc. to encourage spontaneous conversation and discussion.

Lisa's mother talks about the books in their home and Lisa's enjoyment of books and stories, and comments on the fact that Lisa insists on a story at bedtime each night. She also reports that Lisa has always loved books and has always enjoyed quiet activities such as crayoning, etc. Lisa is apparently doing well at school except for the fact that she has been unable to move beyond the first, logographic stage of reading on to a level where the relationship between graphemes and phonemes is established. So you immediately know that your third hypothesis has been refuted.

You find that Lisa is very chatty and you record her speech as she describes her home and her 2-year-old brother. You notice that Lisa still glides her /r/, as her brother's name is Robert, and that she appears to have a fast rate of speech and will occasionally delete weak syllables during stretches of speech. Formal testing on the comprehension tests, which Lisa enjoys, shows no difficulty in grammar but you feel that there appears to be some lack of vocabulary, particularly as her home is obviously a fairly verbal one. So you are forming the impression that your second hypothesis is partially but not fully refuted.

Lisa enjoys rhymes and can say a number of children's rhymes and sing some songs. However, she does find it difficult to pick out the rhyming pair from a selection of pictures. She is very good at 'I spy', showing that she recognizes the onset of words, but is very poor at noticing when the rhyme is the same (unless she can see the words such as look, book, cook). She is caught out when words rhyme but do not look the same (e.g. bought and fort). So you are fairly clear that your first hypothesis is correct and that Lisa has some difficulties at the metaphonological level that are slowing the development of her reading skills.

You are now ready to discuss with Lisa's mother and with her school the area of her difficulties and to decide whether she needs intervention from you, from the special needs department at school or from a combined programme. Further assessment based on what you have found and what all involved – Lisa, her family, the school – have identified will be needed to develop a useful programme of help for Lisa.

This is just one example of hypothesis generation and testing. This process will take place either overtly or covertly throughout your assessment of a client(s). As you gather more information, you will feel confident to ask additional questions of your data and fill in gaps in your knowledge. You are trying to build a whole picture of the person and the situation, and the relationships between these two.

You have now completed the process of data gathering, analysing and evaluating. You have tried to pull together the strands of the information, and you have used models to help organize and visualize what you have seen and heard. As you have proceeded, you have used the known information to help you generate hypotheses about what might be a problem and what might need further assessment. Your next activity will be a consideration of everything that you know and from this you will need to make decisions on what you might be able to offer this client and his or her family.

Decision-making: prognosis and priorities

As mentioned in Chapter 2, decision-making is a complex process that depends on clinical skill and professional experience. However, an inexperienced therapist will have to make decisions and a systematic and considered approach can help in the process. Following most initial contacts, one of the decisions may well be to assess further and this will relieve the pressure of final decisions. However, clients and others will expect some feedback and information and occasionally, as in a triage system, significant decisions have to be taken quickly. If this is the case, more than one professional will be involved and a set of well-defined criteria will be in place to guide you.

Some models of decision-making approaches are pattern recognition, decision trees and decision frameworks.

Pattern recognition

Experienced speech and language clinicians will be able quickly to identify possible areas of difficulty by connecting what they see and hear into patterns. This form of decision-making will be used in a system demanding instant future plans. At an open clinic a clinician may:

- notice that a child of 3 is chewing bricks rather than building with them
- notice that he is not responding to his mother calling his name
- find out from a quick discussion with his mother that he is very quiet and makes his needs known by pointing mostly.

The clinician will hypothesize that this child has possibly a general delay and certainly very delayed language and he or she will decide to book this child in for further assessment. At the same clinic another child is observed:

- He also chews rather than builds the bricks
- He watches the other children intently and looks at the adults as they are speaking about him
- His mother reports that he is saying a lot but it is hard to understand him.

Here the clinician hypothesizes that this child has a delay in speech production that may be phonological or articulatory. He is only just 3 and the clinician gives his mother a home programme related to listening to sounds and plans to see him again in 3 months.

Decision-making tree

An example of a decision-making tree is taken from Chandler and Pickering (2004) (Figure 3.10). They needed to make decisions about managing clinical caseloads in a paediatric community setting. Having analysed what the current situation was and having considered aspects of good practice, they proceeded to define appropriate decisions about intervention based on a number of options as set out in Figure 3.10.

Decision framework

A decision framework is provided by Dodd (1995) to consider systematically the available information and the significance of this. She considers factors in relation to:

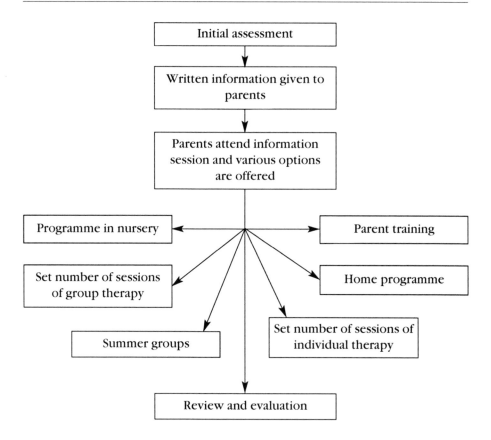

Figure 3.10 A decision-making tree. (From Chandler and Pickering 2004, p. 10.)

- the nature of the language disorder
- severity
- age
- causal and/or maintaining factors.

The nature of the language disorder

There are known characteristics associated with certain disorders that can help you decide what level of outcome is realistic, e.g.:

- A phonological delay affecting only one or two processes is more likely to remediate fully over time than a more pervasive disorder of the sound system.
- A chronic stutter is known to be lasting where a language delay may 'catch up' over time.
- A progressive disorder takes a certain known course, although the timespan differs, whereas an acute acquired difficulty, as a result of, say, a

traumatic brain injury, will have a less predictable outcome dependent on medical and other factors.

Severity

Generally, the more severe a condition, the more difficult and long term will be its remediation. When considering severity, however, you need to ask what you mean by this. Severity must be considered in terms of the impairment, the limitations in activity, and the restriction of participation in general community life that is felt by the client, e.g.:

- The loss of a larynx is very severe, but the likelihood of being able to communicate fully and effectively may be less affected than when the person is aphasic after a stroke.
- Communicative effectiveness would seem to be a good measure of severity, but this would not be the case in, for example, a voice disorder in a professional singer where communication would be unaffected to any major extent but livelihood would be the determining factor.
- An adult who stutters shows a high percentage of dysfluent behaviour with a number of associated movements and a high degree of tension in the musculature. He has a severe stuttering symptom. However, this person holds down a good job, has a family and many friends, and has come to therapy because he is concerned about the effect that his stuttering might have on his young son's speech development. So his needs for therapy would be very different from those of someone who has allowed his stutter to restrict his life considerably.

Age

Age plays a major role in the decision equation. This may be in relation to what services are available to the client depending on his or her age, or it may be about availability or amount of input that is considered appropriate at certain ages. But remember, it is written into the code of practice that you must not discriminate on the grounds of age. If a client appears to need a particular treatment it is morally wrong to withhold it just because the client is very elderly.

Some examples of the significance of the factor of age are:

- Age of onset can give clues as to the nature of the disorder in, for example, children on the autistic spectrum or people who are dysfluent. So you will use the factor of age to help make a differential diagnosis between, for example, a stutter and normal non-fluency.
- The age at which a disorder or delay is identified and intervention is begun are very important, e.g. in hearing loss, stuttering, specific language impairment where it is known that early intervention can prevent some of the more pervasive aspects of the problems developing.

- Intervention before a difficulty is identified in 'at-risk' children is being promoted by a number of managers and clinicians.
- Age of onset of an acquired disorder may have considerable implications both medically and socially, and consequently on possible treatment outcomes. Factors such as general health, possible extension or progression of the complaint, support networks, etc., may be age related.
- Age of the client at this particular point in time will be significant in terms of social, vocational, educational and interpersonal factors, all of which may have an effect on the general motivation of the client.
- Age in relation to length of time since the onset of the condition is important, because, generally, the longer the problem has existed, the more difficult it is likely to be to change.

Causal or maintaining factors

In many of your clients there is no clear cause of their speech or language difficulty. Even where there is an obvious medical cause, as in cancer leading to glossectomy, the environmental maintaining factors in relation to each client will make decision-making different on every occasion. It is acknowledged that most developmental language problems are multicausal, so you need to think broadly of all the possible contributors to the difficulty. Some of these factors may become the focus of your therapy, as, for example, when you decide to work directly with the teachers of a child with pragmatic disorder because you feel that they are unaware of the problem. Others will give some sense of the way in which you may need to offer therapy, e.g. you may offer short-term intensive therapy to a child with phonological delay and her parents because you are aware of the pressure of impending schooling building up in the household. At times, a knowledge of the causal or maintaining factors will lead you to a decision not to intervene, e.g. if a client with advanced multiple sclerosis has reached a life-threatening point and his family do not wish to be 'bothered' by professionals.

Some further examples of the influence of knowledge of these factors in your decision-making are given in Table 3.10.

Working through the process

Case discussions: Adam and Charles

Nature of the language disorder

Both children present with a developmental language delay. Byers Brown and Edwards (1989) suggest that this term, as well as 'developmental language disorder', is used descriptively and is not a diagnostic category itself. It includes children with some known causal factors as well as those with none. The range of language behaviours that the children show is great and

Table 3.10 Structural and functional factors that are significant in causing or maintaining speech and language and swallowing problems

Factor	Decision
Structural differences (e.g. cleft palate)	Remediation may be more long term
Chromosomal differences (e.g. Down's syndrome)	Some intervention may be necessary through lifespan
Brain damage	Full return to pre-morbid state unlikely
Progressive neurological disorder	Deterioration of function, including swallowing, will continue
Sensory loss	May affect nature and timing of intervention
Genetic predisposition or family history (e.g. stammering)	Higher likelihood of becoming chronic
Significant health problems	May affect ability of individual to benefit from intervention
Mother tongue – bilingual and cultural issues	Where and with whom therapy might occur, use of bilingual co-worker or interpreter
Caregiver communication	Language levels, prosody and communicative strategies of others may be focus of intervention
Expectations of others	Demands placed on the individual, needs of others for competence and and 'normal modes of expression' will have to be addressed
School, work, social environments	The effect of these on the difficulties experienced by the client and the role of intervention in education and training
Personal, emotional factors	Awareness and concern of client or others and the impact on communication

difficulties may be seen in comprehension and/or expression in the realms of syntax and/or semantics and/or phonology and/or pragmatics, as well as possible problems with reading and writing.

Severity

Adam presents with no verbal expression. He makes his needs known by pointing and producing a high-pitched [e]. His parents both seem to understand and anticipate his needs and supply him with what he wants almost immediately. On the rare occasions when they are unable to guess, Adam will fling himself on the floor and have a full-blown tantrum wherever he is. His parents try to avoid this as much as possible by always carrying toys and snacks that he enjoys to try to distract him if he looks as if he may be getting frustrated. Adam's parents feel that he understands what they say within reason – he will go and get named items and show interest when they tell him where they are going – but he often appears to ignore what they ask. He plays well with cars, Lego, his bike and a football, but usually requires that his parents play with him. He is an only child.

Charles also has very little verbal expression. He has a few words, recognizable to his parents, for his dog, his favourite toy (a stuffed rabbit) and his bottle, which he takes to bed. His parents describe him as easygoing and no bother. He doesn't seem to need much entertaining and will sit rocking with his rabbit for long periods. He is a fussy eater and his mother gets concerned about this. At present he will eat only bananas and Weetabix. He will suddenly go off these foods and on to another limited set. Charles's parents say that he pays very little attention to them and, while he is fairly compliant if they take him by the hand and lead him to where they want, he does not show much awareness of their language to him. He does, however, enjoy songs and sounds on television. Charles has an older brother with whom he enjoys rough-and-tumble play.

You can begin to organize the information you have obtained so far. By highlighting the importance of the information through +s for significance and −s for insignificance, you can build a picture of their needs that will affect your decision-making (Table 3.11).

Table 3.11 Severity of symptoms for Adam and Charles

Adam		Charles	
Severe symptom –	expression +++ comprehension ++	Severe symptom –	expression +++ comprehension +++
Parental concern +++		Parental concern +	
Child awareness ++		Child awareness –	
Affects family life ++		Affects family life +	

Age

Both boys are 3 years of age. However, there are differences in what might be considered the age of onset when the parents are questioned.

Adam seemed to develop well. He was an alert baby and his motor milestones were within the early normal range: he sat alone at 5 months, was crawling at 7 months and walking at 10 months. He showed an alert interest in everything and made the expected baby cooing and babbling according to his parents. It was not till he was 2 that they began to worry about his lack of words. He had made his needs known so well without words that his parents had not really realized that he was behind until his mother took him to a mother and toddler group. She had expressed some concern to her doctor but was assured that, as everything else was coming along well, Adam would probably catch up in this area.

Charles had always been a good baby. He slept a lot and did not seem to demand food. He was happy to be woken and fed and would look at his mother and smile, but did not seem very interested in anything around him. His parents knew he was very different from their first child and questioned whether he was deaf. When he was 1 year old his doctor arranged for a hearing test. He responded well to visual reinforcement audiometry and he was healthy and developing well, if a little slowly, so his parents were told that there was no problem. At 2 he was saying a few words and, although he was very different from his brother, his parents accepted that he was simply slower in development and were not very concerned. When he was 3, he joined a nursery class and it was there that his lack of language became very apparent.

So, while both boys are showing a definite delay in language, it appears that this is part of a more general developmental delay for Charles. Charles's parents have been aware of a problem from an early age whereas Adam's parents have only really identified a difficulty since language should have been developing (Table 3.12).

Table 3.12 Age as significant for Adam and Charles

Adam	Charles
Child's age +	Child's age +
Time between age noticed and present -	Time between age noticed and present +++

Causal and/or maintaining factors

A few decisions can be made at present based on the information you have about the boys. But there are likely to be many more questions that you will need to ask and observations that you will need to make before you can feel that you know enough to be confident about causal or maintaining factors.

There seem to be few causal factors in Adam's case. His mother had no illnesses during pregnancy and he has had none since. His general development suggests no overt neurological problems and there is no history of speech difficulties in the family. Adam sees well and his parents feel that he hears well. A simple speech discrimination test suggests that he is hearing sounds distinctively and you are not overly concerned about his hearing although you will keep an eye on this and refer him for a full hearing test if you feel that it is necessary at a later date. The environmental factors that are significant are the amount of concern expressed by his parents and the fact that Adam can obtain his needs without speech. He shows an obvious awareness and sensitivity to communication breakdown and is already manipulating his parents through his tantrums. Adam seems to be able in many areas: he plays symbolically and imaginatively, he is keen to group and match, and plays simple games of snap and pelmanism. In fact he is very capable of recalling what pictures he has recently turned over. As a result of his severe expressive language difficulty, his parents don't know whether he can recall auditory information such as nursery rhymes but his mother reports that he can anticipate the actions in rhymes such as 'Ring-o-Roses'. Adam attends a nursery three afternoons a week where he seems to play well with other children.

Charles has a very different pattern from Adam. His mother reported a series of minor ailments during the pregnancy and an increase in blood pressure leading to inducement of the birth a week before the due date. Charles had been a good size but was slow to breathe and was in a special baby unit for a day. After that he picked up and did well. He was always a slow feeder and was often sick, but he put on weight slowly and went home from hospital a week after his birth. While he had never had any major illnesses, he often had colds and chestiness. He sat at 10 months, did not crawl but pulled himself about from 1 year. He walked at 18 months and since then has progressed well on gross motor skills. His hearing is of concern, even though he passed the early test. There is no history of speech problems in the family and his brother is doing well and has no difficulties. Environmental factors are the lack of expectations of him in the home. Charles is somewhat repetitive in his play. He enjoys grouping and sorting objects but will do this to the exclusion of other activities. His brother says he will not play a card game with him, nor will Charles play imaginatively. He does enjoy football and running around outside, however. At nursery he is very active and enjoys the climbing frame and the bikes, but the nursery teachers find it difficult to contain him during quieter activities such as painting or stories.

There are now additional factors to add to the strengths and areas of difficulty of the two boys (Table 3.13), and you have reached a point where you need to use the information gathered in order to reach a decision about future management. Your options are:

- to do nothing
- to refer on
- to give a home programme
- to see for review at a later date
- to offer indirect therapy via others
- to offer direct therapy with parents only or child only
- to offer direct therapy with child and parents together
- to see for therapy occasionally
- to see for therapy regularly.

Collation of all the information known so far about Adam and Charles

You now need to work through a process of considering the significance of the information that you have collected. You might start by asking yourself questions and following the answers through in a logical step-by-step fashion.

Table 3.13 Causative and maintenance factors for Adam and Charles

Adam	Charles
Pregnancy factors –	Pregnancy factors +
Past illnesses –	Past illnesses ++
Neurological factors:	Neurological factors:
attention –	attention ++
listening skills +	listening skills +++
memory/learning skills –	memory/learning skills ++
development –	development +
sensory –	sensory ++
family history –	family history –
Environment:	Environment:
parental concern +++	parental concern –
child awareness ++	child awareness –

Question 1: Is there cause for concern in the areas investigated?

General summary of the two children (Table 3.14)

Adam's language difficulty seems to be more specifically focused on verbal expression than Charles's. Parental anxiety is the major area of concern in relation to maintaining factors, but Adam also shows a high degree of awareness and reaction to his difficulties. Although Adam is still only 3, his communicative behaviour is similar to that of a 12- to 18-month-old child, so it is severely delayed.

Charles's problem seems to be more pervasive and affects many more cognitive areas of behaviour than Adam's. His comprehension of language appears to be minimal and his lack of interest in communication is of concern. Charles appears to have some causative areas of significance pointing to possible neurological dysfunction.

Table 3.14 Collation of all the information about Adam and Charles

Area of concern	Adam	Charles
Language expression	+++	+++
Language comprehension	++	+++
Parental concern	+++	+
Child awareness	++	
Family life affected	++	+
Development		+
Pregnancy		+
Illnesses		+
Attention		++
Listening skill	+	+++
Memory/learning skills		++
Sensory		++
Family history		

Both children have interested and involved parents and both are of similar age.

Decisions and prognoses

Following this careful consideration of the data, you can now start to make some decisions about which options to follow. You may first consult the criteria for prioritization and caseload management that is in use in your work context. Thus you may rate Adam and Charles in terms of:

1. Communication skills in relation to other skills
   0 communication skills commensurate with other level of skill
   1 communication skills slightly delayed compared to other levels of skill
   2 communication skills significantly delayed compared to other levels of skill
   Adam 2; Charles 1

2. Severity of communication difficulty
   0 slight impairment to communication
   1 slight-to-moderate impairment
   2 severe communication difficulty
   Adam 2; Charles 2

3. Readiness for intervention
   0 not ready
   1 just ready
   2 very ready
   Adam 2; Charles 0/1

4. Potential for change
   0 poor potential
   1 moderate potential
   2 good potential
   Adam 2; Charles 1

5. Client/carer anxiety
   0 little anxiety
   1 moderately anxious
   2 very anxious
   Adam 2; Charles 0

It is already becoming apparent that the priorities for these two boys are different. You now consider your options for intervention:

• to offer information/home programme for parents

- to offer information/programme/support for others
- to offer a group for the child only or for the parents only
- to offer a group for the parents and child to attend together
- to offer individual therapy for child only or parents only
- to offer individual therapy with child and parents together
- to see intensively, or occasionally (e.g. every month)
- to see for a specific period (e.g. 4 weeks, 6 weeks) or unspecified.

You decide that:

1. Both children need some kind of intervention as their language delay is severe.
2. Adam is higher on the priority list for immediate intervention than Charles.
3. Both need their hearing checked although there is more concern in Charles's case because of a lack of response to his parents' language.
4. Both sets of parents are keen to be involved and home programmes of listening skills (for Adam) and attention and listening (for Charles) will be given.
5 As Adam is showing frustration and developing behavioural responses to his difficulty, and as his parents show a high level of concern, a parent–child non-directive approach will be taken based on the parent–child interaction therapy of Rustin et al. (1996).
6. Charles has just started nursery and you realize that a collaborative programme with staff is essential. You feel that Charles may have a more general delay and may be exhibiting some signs of a pragmatic disorder. You decide to see him on a fortnightly basis while he is settling in and, with his parents' permission, will ask a colleague experienced in autistic spectrum disorder to observe him.
7. You suggest a summer group of listening and attention for Charles. For Adam, a group needs to be considered carefully because it could encourage him to be more outgoing or undermine his self-esteem even more.

This same careful analysis of information can be applied to any person with any disorder and leads to decisions that are based on knowledge and facts. Other factors may, of course, be part of the equation, such as the policy of your employer, the nature of your timetable, the ability of other professionals to be involved, and so on.

As you become involved with the client (in this case the child and his family) you need to adjust flexibly to what you are learning through the ongoing process of assessment and reassessment, negotiation with those involved and the outcomes your intervention is aimed towards.

Having discussed the process of assessment and decision-making in detail, in Chapter 4 we go on to consider the process of therapy. This moves on from the base of the hypotheses and decisions made but keeps returning to these and to the whole assessment process as a means of checking its effectiveness and direction. The purpose of assessment is discovery whereas the purpose of therapy is to bring about change. Change will lead to new discoveries, so while therapy is being undertaken, assessment and the gaining of information and knowledge will be continuing hand in hand.

Chapter 4
Therapy: process and practice

You sit on the floor with a child and from a big bag you pull interesting objects that you then cause to disappear under a cloth, only to make them re-emerge and jump into the child's hand. As you do this you make the noise of the object – a chuffing train, a whistling bird, a buzzing bee. The child delightedly hides the objects behind his back and you pretend to look for them. You 'call' each item by making its noise. You then find the items behind the child, who laughs and gives them up as you hold out your hand and make the noise for each. Is this therapy?

You sit at a table in your clinic with a child and her mother. You put on the table a series of pictures and encourage the child to find the sequence that tells the story. You then ask the child to tell her mother the story. As the three of you work together on this, you comment on the pictures that the child seems to find difficult: 'Oh, this is where they are packing to go on holiday. I can see dad putting the case in the car.' You remind the child of aspects of the pictures that she has missed, not in a judgemental way but in a way designed to engage her interest in providing information: 'Did you tell your mother about the dog jumping into the car?' (said quietly so the information is not yet shared by the child's mother). Is this therapy?

You sit quietly in a room next to an elderly woman. She is trying to tell you about her son who has moved to another town. She makes many false starts, she chooses and rejects the words or sounds that make up the words that she is trying to utter. She gestures and points. You feed back what you have heard; you ask for more information about the place; you follow her pointing hand and suggest an area of the country it might be in; you offer a phoneme as a cue for a town in that locality. Eventually, she is able to produce a word close enough to the name of a town where you know he is living. You comment on her persistence and her ability to get the information across and she looks relieved and more relaxed. Is this therapy?

Defining therapy

What has been described above can be loosely termed 'methods'. Methods are what you do but they do not by themselves constitute therapy. So what is

96

therapy? Byng and Black (1995, p. 305) suggest that in language remediation therapy is 'a combination of the task, the materials and the psycholinguistic concepts conveyed through the task, and the therapist/patient interaction'. To try to understand what therapy is composed of, you may find the iceberg model shown in Figure 4.1 helpful.

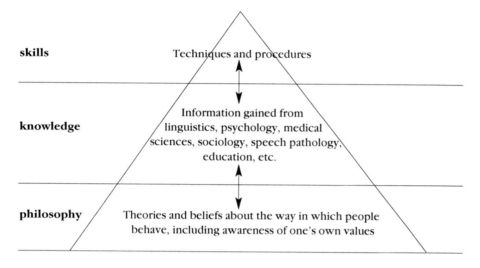

skills Techniques and procedures

knowledge Information gained from linguistics, psychology, medical sciences, sociology, speech pathology, education, etc.

philosophy Theories and beliefs about the way in which people behave, including awareness of one's own values

Figure 4.1 A model for defining therapy. (After Stengelhofen, 1993.)

The pinnacle of this iceberg, the *skills* level, is the techniques and procedures such as those described earlier. These are on the surface and are those aspects of the process seen by others. Comments from those who do not understand the profession, such as 'Oh, anyone can talk to an old lady' or 'Why do you need a degree to teach you to play with children?', stem from an ignorance of what is under the surface of the water, of what underpins procedures that look so easy.

The next level under that of skills, and from which skills evolve, is that of *knowledge*. It is impossible to decide what you should do with a person in therapy without a sound knowledge of the linguistic and other difficulties that are present, the approaches recommended in the literature for understanding and treating these disorders, and the developmental and psychological factors inherent in the person who is in therapy. You develop your competence in this area from the linguistics, medical sciences, psychology, sociology, education and speech pathology that you learn as part of your university training.

The deepest level of the iceberg is that of *philosophy*. Your decisions about how you will use your knowledge and develop techniques of therapy are driven by your thinking about how people learn, what motivates them, how they come to see the world as they do, why they behave in certain ways. Equally important are your own beliefs and values and how they influence your actions and decisions.

Based on this model, therapy can be defined as behaviours that come about through a combination of philosophy, knowledge and skills, all three of which influence and are influenced by the others through processes of monitoring and of reflection.

The levels of the therapy process

We now look more closely at each of the three levels of the therapy process, starting with the deepest and least obvious level, that of philosophy. This is the level that can so often be unrecognized and neglected, and yet it may drive decisions and procedures. It must therefore be made explicit so that it can be used purposefully in therapeutic decision-making.

Philosophy

1. Observation and imitation, modelling of behaviour, feedback, reinforcement, reward and punishment are all based on the idea that behaviour can be learned when it has certain consequences, and a therapist can aid or manipulate this learning by carefully monitoring and contingently reacting to a client's behaviour. The principles of *learning theory*, and particularly of *behaviourism,* have had an enormous influence on the profession and the therapy that is offered. Your decisions about whether or not to adopt a teaching role, how structured or unstructured your therapy programme will be and how to manage issues of general behaviour will most likely stem from your awareness and utilization of learning theory.
2. Attitudes and beliefs, values and prejudice, and the influence of these on learning and thinking and on the way people behave form the basis of *cognitive theories* that underlie many of the techniques that you might use to help your clients develop realistic self-awareness.
3. A belief in the capability of your client to change and develop, to make decisions and to come to his or her own solutions, as well as approaches that enhance your client's self-esteem and realistic self-concept, will be based on your own understanding of theories of personality, particularly those of the *humanistic school.* Decisions about how much to involve your client as a partner in the therapeutic process and how directive or non-directive your approaches will be may stem from this underlying philosophy.
4. An awareness of the influence of society and of various groups and interpersonal relationships on an individual's behaviour, and an understanding of contexts and their influence on behaviour, form the basis of *social theories* that drive decisions about where and with whom therapy will take place. *Social constructionism* alerts the therapist to the power of

language and the ways in which society constructs views about health and illness, which then influence policy and thought.

5. The idea of the person as individually making sense of his or her own experience is the basis of *contructivism*. When you acknowledge that your client's view of his condition is 'real' to him and is linked to the way in which he sees himself and others and his world, and you listen credulously without judgement to what he is saying you are working within the frame of personal construct theory (Kelly 1955).

6. The need of all of us to organize and structure our experiences, to convey them in an orderly form and to have someone listen to what we have to say about ourselves is acknowledged by *narrative* theory which has emerged from constructivist/constructionist and systems theories (McLeod 1997).

There are probably many more underlying philosophies that direct and influence the behaviour of the therapist and his or her understanding of the people with whom therapy will be conducted. Those outlined above have all had a clear influence over the years on the way speech and language therapy is conducted. Certain philosophies hold sway at certain times – they grow out of the knowledge, beliefs and expectations of the society in which you live. You must remember that much of your perception of human behaviour is based on western European ideals and must be critically examined when it conflicts with the philosophies of clients who may come from other cultural and social backgrounds. Philosophical concepts and ideas are open to modification and change as new knowledge and new beliefs emerge.

Knowledge

In previous chapters, the areas of knowledge that are used as the basis of exploration and understanding of the speech and language difficulties that affect clients have been discussed. Gaining and stabilizing this knowledge will form a major part of your student years. Knowledge does not exist in a vacuum, it is integrated with your clinical reasoning and it is moulded and used in different ways depending on your clients, your environments and your aims. Knowledge is transferable. This is important to remember and can reduce the pressure of the need to know everything in every setting! What you learn about language disorder in adults can be used in relation to children with some adjustments. An understanding of the symptoms of a fluency disorder or the medical reasons for a voice disorder can be applied across all ages, e.g.:

> Mr Jones has had a stroke. He has aphasia and has particular difficulty in saying what he wants – he cannot find the words. Joe is 8 years and in a mainstream school. He has a language disorder and finds it hard to choose the vocabulary needed to express himself. What do you need to know in order to come to decisions about therapy for Mr Jones and for Joe?

1. You need knowledge from medical texts. This will help you understand the reason for Mr Jones' particular language problems – how these relate to the location of his brain damage and the functions that this location generally controls. For Joe, you will learn about family history of speech and language disorders and the possible genetic links with these. A sound understanding of the neurophysiological underpinnings of speech and language disorders will be learned from texts such as that of Atkinson and McHanwell (2002).

2. You will gain much of your understanding of the problems that affect Mr Jones and Joe from the area of linguistics. People who have problems 'finding' words are experiencing difficulties in learning or in retrieving the lexical item that represents the particular thing, e.g. Joe, in trying to explain that he has seen a swan, may be unable to visualize the creature sufficiently well to put a name to it, whereas Mr Jones (who prior to his stroke could easily name a swan) will probably have a clear image of the bird but he will find it hard to retrieve the correct form of the word 'swan' from his memory (Marshall 1998). It is essential for a speech and language clinician to have a good knowledge of how people learn and use words, constructing them out of a sequence of correct sounds that make up the words, and placing these into sentences to convey meaning to others. This can be gained only through study of linguistics and phonetics (see books such as that by Black and Chiat 2003).

3. We have touched on the aspect of memory and how words and sounds need to be retrieved from a memory store of some kind. Understanding why Mr Jones cannot recall the word 'swan' or why Joe cannot remember enough about the bird in order to name it requires knowledge of aspects of the functioning brain such as perception, attention and memory. Details of these will be found in texts on cognitive psychology such as that by Eysenck (2001). The field of knowledge that tries to work out the way that language is processed by the brain is that of psycholinguistics. Psycholinguists construct models of the working brain, trying to understand how 'errors' of understanding or production of language may occur (Ellis and Young 1998). As a speech and language clinician, you need to understand the cognitive/processing level at which difficulty arises for a person like Mr Jones or a child like Joe in order that you may target these areas in your therapy. Books such as those by Rapp (2001) and Stackhouse and Wells (1997) help you to understand and apply this knowledge to your clients.

4. Mr Jones finds that he can recall the word 'swan' on some occasions and not on others. Similarly Joe has been heard to use the word 'swan' before. Why is it that the word seems to come and go? Here your knowledge needs to broaden into areas of sociology or education to try to understand the effect that social pressure or educational programmes may have on your two clients. You should also be interested in the effect that this diffi-culty in communication might have on Mr Jones and Joe as individuals or

on the people who relate to Mr Jones or Joe (Brumfitt 1999). If you know about social stigma and the way in which different cultures or social groups might react to impairments, you can better understand the activity limitations and restrictions on participation that being unable to say what you want when you want may impose on Mr Jones and Joe. You must also be aware of the implications of your own interactions with Mr Jones or Joe and the imbalance in language knowledge and use between clinician and client which can detract from rather than facilitate improvement in your clients (Ferguson and Armstrong 2004).

5. Finally, you will want to have a sound knowledge of speech and language therapy in order to make clinical decisions and find appropriate and effective therapy tasks for Mr Jones and Joe. For Mr Jones you might embark on the use of cueing as a therapy tool to aid his retrieval of words (Best et al. 1998). Numerous books and articles are published on the area of therapy. Joe may well respond to work on Semantic Links (Bigland and Speake 1992) and/or a Metaphon approach to aid his storage of word forms (Howell and Dean 1994). It is important that you read a number of these rather than simply grasp at the first one you come across. Remember, it is your duty as a professional to choose the approach that is most effective according to experts in the field.

These, and other, approaches are available for you as a therapist to use, and the more you know and understand the various philosophies underlying them and the skills and procedures of which they are composed, the wider will be your choice. Your decision about which approach to choose should be based on what you and your client have agreed seems to be best at this time. It may be that your basic underlying philosophy will sway you towards a particular approach. You must ask yourself 'Is this the right one for this person at this time?' Only your knowledge of yourself, your client and the options available can prevent you from making the wrong choice of therapy. But sometimes you just will not know whether this client will respond to a certain kind of approach. In such cases, careful explanation of why you are trying a certain approach and what criteria you will use to decide whether to proceed or to change it is necessary. Remember that a hypothesis-driven approach is necessary in therapy – 'If we try X then Y should happen'. If it does not happen, then a new hypothesis is in order. Many therapy practices that work well arise out of cautious trial-and-error approaches.

Skills

When you see someone who is very skilled working, you will often exclaim at how easy it all looks. The session flows smoothly, the client is engaged and interested, the tasks are meaningful in relation to the client's age, sex, culture, disability, etc. What skills are being used? Stengelhofen (1993) suggests that the skills shown in Figure 4.2 are important in clinical management.

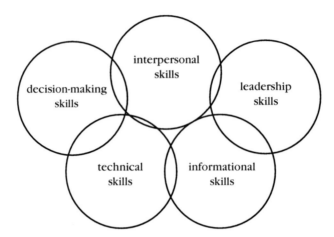

Figure 4.2 Skills in clinical management. The skills are represented as overlapping circles to suggest that, although they may be defined separately, they depend on and support each other. (After Stengelhofen, 1993.)

Similarly Parker and Kersner (2001) suggest that there are five key skills needed to work effectively as a speech and language clinician:

1. Interpersonal skills
2. Information-gathering skills
3. Therapy skills
4. Problem-solving and decision-making skills
5. Organizational skills.

The following discussion is based on an integration of the ideas of these authors and ourselves.

Decision-making and problem-solving skills

In Chapter 3, we discussed decision-making skills in relation to whether or not to offer therapy. In this chapter, we are interested in how a task is chosen. Remember that the choice of task must be based on the aims and objectives for this client. Once you have decided these (which we look at later in this chapter), the skill of planning the task is embarked upon:

• You might see a therapist engaged in tasks with a child and parent, such as blowing bubbles through a straw, playing with a toy garage and cars, arranging pictures into a sequence and retelling the story.
• You may see him or her having a conversation, asking the client to think of as many items within one semantic category as possible within a time limit or drawing pictures of items to be bought in a shop.

- The therapist might be engaging a group in a game of 'wink murder', asking members to solve a problem together or planning and going ahead with an outing of some kind.

How is the therapist making decisions about what activities to do in therapy? How has he or she decided whether to see this client individually or in a group or with the family? How has the clinician decided to do this activity at this moment and how will she decide when to move on or change tasks? To make these decisions you might need to be competent at the skills shown in Figure 4.3, for example.

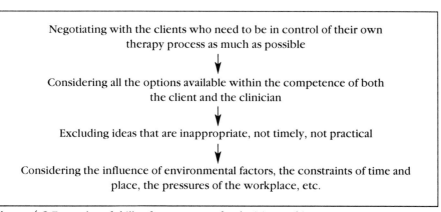

Figure 4.3 Examples of skills of competency for decision-making.

Interpersonal skills

Developing a good rapport, being sensitive to the client's needs, knowing when fatigue or emotion are taking over and how to deal with them when they do, knowing how to alter the pace, tone or level of the activity are all part of being competent in the area of interpersonal skills. Dryden (1990) asked authorities in counselling what qualities an effective therapist needs within the therapy regimen offered by a particular approach. Many of these authors agreed that the qualities were:

- the core counselling qualities of genuineness, warmth and empathy, which are based on the skills of observing, listening and responding appropriately
- sensitivity to others
- respect for clients
- a credulous approach (i.e. accept what the client offers as truth for him or her)
- self-awareness
- a desire to go on developing and broadening life experiences
- trustworthiness and dependability.

Therapeutic relationships are built and sustained through informed involvement of the therapist. They do not just 'happen'. You have to work hard to reach a competent level in the ability to build rapport with clients.

Another set of interpersonal skills that are constantly in use by the speech and language clinician is those loosely termed 'social skills'. These are based on a sensitivity to what is appropriate in a given situation and knowing how to modify your own behaviour when in this situation. So you might:

- adopt a quiet listening role when negotiating how a teacher might help a child in his or her classroom, adapting your posture, facial expressions and proximity to convey the acceptance of the teacher's dominant role in classroom management
- be assertive and confident when providing models of therapy techniques to clients and their carers in the clinic using clear speech, adequate volume and well-controlled gestures and movements
- be calm and slow-moving when presented with a highly anxious individual, reducing eye contact and keeping a fair distance from the client so as not to be seen as a threat
- show enthusiasm and excitement when playing a game with a child, getting on the same physical level as the child, and using a lot of eye contact, facial expression and increased intonation
- adopt the rules of reduced eye contact or increased formality that are expected when with a client from a different cultural background.

As you can see, the ability to modify behaviours such as facial expression, proximity, etc. in appropriate ways is directly related to the development of the core qualities as specified by Dryden above. In addition, as speech and language clinicians we need (see Parker and Kersner 2001, for additional information):

- good expressive communication skills such as oral skills that are adapted to the language needs of our clients
- the ability to sign or use symbols or electronic aids
- a core skill, which is the ability to explain, demonstrate and present information and ideas to our clients effectively
- the skills of collaborating in order to work effectively with clients and all other interested parties. This implies a developing understanding of the need to break down the imbalance of therapist as communicative expert and client as container of communication difficulties (see the clinical forum on speech and language therapists' talk introduced by Ferguson and Armstrong (2004) and debated by a number of other contributors).

Leadership and organizational skills

These two skills are being combined because, in order to be a good leader, it is essential that you manage yourself and your work life effectively. You need to be able to take the initiative, make choices, act on decisions and move things forward or you will never cope with the workaday life of a speech and language clinician. Managing your time and your workload, knowing when to ask for help and when to 'go it alone', and knowing how and when to follow procedures are part of the Health Profession Council's (HPC's) expectations of you as an autonomous and accountable professional (HPC 2003). As a leader of numerous different groups, you need to know how and when to direct, facilitate or guide groups of people as you teach skills, or enable group dynamics to emerge, or encourage joint learning. Fawcus (1992) reminds us that, whether or not we take account of the psychosocial factors in a group, the mere fact of being part of a group will have a positive or negative effect on the attitudes and feelings of the participants. It is very important therefore that you know and understand what the dynamics of groups are and what role you will play as leader.

Technical skills

What are the technical skills of a speech and language clinician? In our profession they are less easy to identify and isolate than in some other professions where particular accurate measures might be relatively straightforward, e.g. measuring the length of one leg against another, or the height:weight ratio of a person, etc. Below we have identified a few of the technical skills in speech and language therapy, but you could probably add many, many more:

- Measurement in speech and language therapy requires a knowledge of the standardized, or preferred, way of administering a procedure and the standard way of recording the information. So reading and understanding manuals associated with testing procedures would be a way of acquiring this skill.
- Manipulation of the switches on a recording device and understanding how to get the best audio or video recording (taking into account light, ambient noise, etc.) are important skills.
- Transcription of linguistic information in a standard form – using conventions for orthographic or phonetic transcription – is a very skilled job based on much practice.
- Management of the testing or teaching equipment in the therapy space, so that it is accessible but not distracting, helps the ease and flow of the therapy session.
- Choosing, making or adapting materials to suit the client(s) and their level of ability is a skill based on a strong knowledge base.
- Modelling wanted behaviours, and cueing and reinforcing to channel or modify clients' attempts to reach a planned goal, are skills based on knowledge of goal-setting and behaviour modification.
- Using counselling skills such as attending behaviours, paraphrasing, reflecting, summarizing, etc., to encourage clients to feel able to discuss information openly.

- Recording behaviour and activities as they occur in the therapy sessions, and use of appropriate and relatively quick scoring methods to keep records of outcomes of your interventions, is a vital skill, again based on knowledge of anticipated goals.

Informational skills

When you meet a client or his family, the teacher of a child with speech and language difficulties or a voluntary group wanting to know and understand the nature of language problems, you need to call on the skills of gathering and giving information. When you write a report or give verbal feedback on a client, or you plan a programme with a teacher or prepare a workshop session for a group of care workers, you need to draw on skills of preparing and presenting visual information. So you need to develop:

- a good level of knowledge in the particular area
- an ability to present this knowledge in a 'user-friendly' fashion
- a sensitivity to the level of language needed
- good on-line recording of information
- an ability to provide information in ways that are sensitive to client needs, e.g. in a different language or in symbol form
- an awareness of adult learning styles and the way in which your information giving is being received and responded to.

Heron (1990) suggests that there is a directive continuum along which any prescriptive intervention (which is what information giving is) can be placed. This has five grades from mild to strong: (1) suggest, (2) propose, (3) advise, (4) persuade and (5) command.

Your own awareness of the 'tone' in which you offer information is essential if you wish clients and others to listen to, remember and respond to what you have to offer.

The therapy plan

Armed with your philosophy, knowledge and skills, you are now ready to start the process of converting theory into practice via the therapy plan. Byng et al. (2000) remind us that the speech and language clinician must be aware of a multiplicity of factors when considering a management plan. The clinician must take into account 'resource issues, the personality of the aphasic person or therapist, their priorities, their health beliefs, the complexities of their immediate social environment, family dynamics and crises, ongoing life events and financial uncertainty'. (Byng et al. are writing about people with aphasia, but their comments can apply to any client with any disorder.) The plan forms a blueprint for the activities that you and your client will undertake to achieve some specified ends. Working without a plan would be a bit like trying to make a dress without a pattern or to build a block of flats with no instructions, measurements or decisions about materials needed! To plan competently, you need a framework similar to the one presented in Figure 4.4. The words used in this flowchart may differ for different people, e.g. the word 'goal' may be used instead of 'objective' and so on, but the principles will be universal.

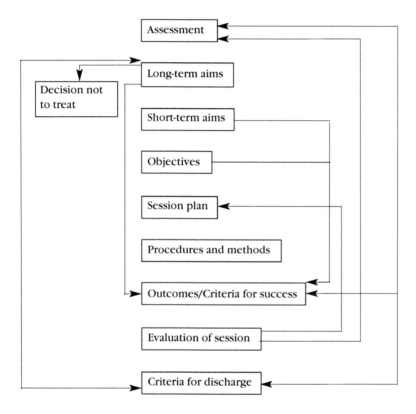

Figure 4.4 A flowchart of the therapy-planning process.

Assessment has a chapter of its own because it is so important (see Chapter 3). It is the starting point for your plan, but also a point to which you constantly return. Therapy can proceed successfully only if you are regularly using what you are learning about the client to review and reconsider the original decisions that you made about his or her difficulties.

Long-term aims/intentions are based on what you know from the assessment and what this tells you about where the client might be at the point of discharge. This requires an understanding of the nature of the condition and its likely course, and factors that lie within the domain of the client (e.g. age, personality and support from others, which were discussed at length in the section on decision-making). It also requires knowledge of the constraints of working practice and practical details, such as availability of transport, distance of the clinic from the client's home, space, time available, etc. For some clients you will be aiming to develop language skills to a level where they are age-appropriate, whereas with others you will hope for communicative competence within the constraints mentioned above. For some you might be looking to maintain skills for as long as possible and offering alternatives when necessary; for yet others you will be providing carers with as much information and support as possible to deal with the long-term language problems presented by their spouse, relative or friend.

These long-term *intentions* would be written as a list of hoped-for outcomes from the point of view of both the clinician and the client. These will be in the areas of impairment, activity limitation, participation restriction and distress at the point when the service user will leave therapy. Together you may hope for:

- specific linguistic changes or other behavioural changes in aspects of reading and writing or play
- changes in access to the curriculum at school or integrating into a community venture of some kind
- changes in motivation to be more active in leisure pursuits or learning
- changes in family or group relationships
- changes in personal and emotional well-being of the clients/users.

Short-term aims will relate directly to the long-term aims but will 'chunk' the timescale of treatment into manageable pieces and will identify where the therapist and client will hope to be within a certain short timescale, such as 6 weeks, 4 weeks, or a school term or semester. You will need to decide what are the priorities for work at this particular time based on the long-term, hoped-for outcomes. These will be negotiated with your client, his or her family, the teaching staff, the ward staff or involved others – you cannot make these decisions on your own. So you will take one or two of the above list and reduce the overall aim into a sequence of sub-aims.

Each set of short-term aims should hopefully be a step up the ladder to the long-term outcomes. The end of the period assigned to reach the short-term aims will be a time for reflecting on progress so far and recycling back to additional assessment or exploration of the problem if necessary.

Objectives or goals are the more tangible outcomes – the actual behaviours or feelings or attitudes – that may change in the process of therapy. They are the carefully analysed sequence of steps that will guide the client to the outcome.

Case discussion: Peter

Peter is a 40-year-old man who was head injured in a fall. He has particular difficulty in maintaining a steady rate of speech. With excessive speed comes elision of syllables and, at times, whole words, which makes Peter very difficult to understand. He is having difficulty monitoring this behaviour. Your short-term aim in relation to this linguistic problem is to improve Peter's ability to recognize fast and unintelligible speech.

Aim

To improve Peter's monitoring skills by helping him recognize when his speech has become very fast.

Objectives

That Peter will:

- learn to use a word-per-minute count to measure rate of speech
- discriminate fast and slow speech of a variety of speakers via tape recordings with 100 per cent accuracy
- identify which of his own spoken sentences are fast, using tape recordings of his speech
- measure his own rate of speech.

At the end of the period of therapy, you should be able to agree with Peter that these objectives have or have not been met and decide what to focus on next.

Session plan

Some examples of session plans are given at the end of this chapter. The session plan starts with the aims and objectives for the particular day, which will be based on the short-term aims and even more precise and detailed than those suggested above. The session plan contains a list of the actual procedures that you will undertake which move the process from the idea to the action. It will also contain suggestions for methods and materials needed to accomplish the procedures.

Procedures are the course of action that will turn the concepts of goals or objectives into tangible activities. Procedures are not arbitrary; they are in fact tightly tied to the aims and objectives and as such are not simply intuitive or random. However, the procedures are the aspect of the therapy process that can be called 'creative'. When a therapist is working well with a client or group of clients, using his or her knowledge and skills effectively, and is sure and clear about the underlying philosophy that is driving the process, we are likely to say that what we are seeing is a very *creative* person.

But what is creativity? De Bono (1985), in interviews with creative people from many walks of life, found that there are numerous different ways of allowing creative ideas to evolve. Among them are the following (for additional information and ideas on creativity see books such as that by Sternberg 1999):

- Put everything you know into 'the pot' (your mind, a piece of paper, a discussion with a colleague), and through this process of brainstorming ideas will evolve.
- Allow yourself to be completely preoccupied with the ideas in order to arrive at solutions.
- Put the knowledge and information you have into groups and categories and take note of any gaps.
- Think freely and widely – what do you still need to know? What approaches would be possible given this client's age, interests, linguistic level, home situation? What are your own biases in therapy and are you being influenced by these? What ideas and suggestions have been given to you by others? What therapy ideas have you read about that might be useful here?

This process of thinking loosely and allowing all thoughts to be accepted and considered is the best way to come to that point of 'Eureka', where you suddenly get an idea or see much more clearly where you are going.

Case discussion: George

Imagine you are faced with the need to develop some tasks in order to meet the objective that your client George, a 60 year old who has aphasia, will begin to initiate more conversation.

Experiences

First, you may think about your own experiences in initiating conversations. What makes it easy or difficult to start? What do you do when you enter a conversation? How do other people that you know initiate conversations? Have you seen other people of this age or other people with aphasia in conversation? How do they cope?

Knowledge

Next you might look at the linguistic literature on conversational exchange to see what is known about the processing needed to initiate language and the skills used to start conversations. You may wish to read the neuropsychological literature to find out what is known about the effects of brain injury on initiation of behaviour. You now turn to your knowledge of this particular man. What is the extent and location of his brain injury? How severe is his linguistic loss? What was he like before the stroke? Did he enjoy and engage in conversation? Who does he have to talk to now? Does this person enjoy and want to be engaged in conversation? What are the hurdles that he will need to overcome if he is to participate in conversation with another?

Perception

The way you look at and make sense of this information is biased by your own experiences and values. You perceive the problem in a particular way. The more you can be aware of and avoid thinking in a channelled fashion, the more creative will be your ideas. You might wish to share ideas for therapy for this man with a friend. Ask questions of your friend as if she were the client. 'How would you feel if I asked you to tell me about your family? What would you do in a situation where you had to engage a stranger in conversation?'

Remember that there are no rights or wrongs in this sort of decision-making. There are a number of alternative procedures that you and your client are free to try out. Once you have embarked on the tasks, you are still not bound to carry them through to the bitter end. Think of yourself and your client as scientists formulating and testing out new hypotheses about what does and does not work, about what might be useful in generating change (Kelly 1963).

Methods and materials

Each step of your overall session plan takes the process to a more micro-scopic level. Methods may be seen therefore as an orderly set of actions based on the overall procedure. Within the method, adjustments of the actions may be written down to enable you to provide more or less support or challenge for the client as appropriate.

Case discussion: George (continued)

Objectives for a session with George

By the end of this session George will have:
• gained my attention by any means possible at least four times
• produced some 'opening' utterance or gesture on each occasion.

Procedures

1. Explain the nature of the task to George.
2. Look at the articles on gardening that he said he would bring.
3. Wait – do not ask questions. This is to give George time to initiate.
4. Respond immediately to any attention-getting device – George might point, move the paper, produce a non-verbal sound (throat-clearing).
5. Respond appropriately to any initiations made by George and paraphrase any verbal attempts.
6. Record George's behaviour and discuss this with him.

Methods

The numbering applies to the procedure to which these methods are attached:

1. Explanation must:
   - focus on idea of starting off
   - reinforce idea that he is more knowledgeable than I am in this area
   - reinforce that he can indicate need for help if necessary.
2. Read a paragraph from one of the articles aloud to focus George's attention:
   - if paragraph seems too difficult produce easier/shorter one
   - if George needs more attention focus, provide additional passage for him to follow as I read.
3. Use non-verbal reinforcements to encourage him to find something to which he wishes to draw my attention (nod, smile, indicate page).
4. If he seems unable to start a conversation, consider:
   - guiding his hand to a point on the page
   - underlining the main points on the page
   - giving alternatives - 'this or this'
   - asking direct questions if he is not forthcoming
   - if he finds it easy, move on to general gardening topics, i.e. remove the visual prompt provided by the articles.
5. Reinforce by continuing on topic that he has introduced, by paraphrasing what he has said, or by giving a general comment on the area that he has indicated.

As you can see the methods are far more detailed than the procedures. It is recommended that you use this level of detail if you are insecure about what you are doing. As you become more confident, you can reduce the detail and write procedures and not methods. Experienced clinicians will be able to carry a set of aims and objectives in their heads and the procedures will come automatically as the session unfolds.

One of the outcomes of carefully thinking about methods is the development of *flexibility*. This means the ability to adapt and respond, relative to the immediate needs of the client. As you can see from the examples above, method 4 gives a range of prompts to use if George is having difficulties and an idea for moving to more spontaneous conversation should he find the task easy. To be flexible you need therefore to have a good understanding of the steps that you will take to reach the goal and the prompts and cues that are appropriate and necessary to get there. You must also have a good idea of what is next in line in the overall programme (the short- and long-term aims and objectives) so you can move up a level if necessary. Every clinician will have experienced times when a client has shown such variability that an impossible task one week is completed with ease the following week. Building flexibility into the methods is the way for an inexperienced clinician to deal with this.

Materials

Materials would appear to be straightforward, but of course they are not. George has said he would bring some gardening articles with him. But what if he forgets? And what will you do about his poor eyesight? Where will you position the magazine to accommodate his inclination to neglect one side? A young child in therapy will need materials that will gain his or her interest, or make the appropriate sounds that are not in any way ambiguous. You will have to arrange to have other distractions out of sight, to reduce noise levels, etc. Will you need a video for work with a mother? Will you ask her to play with her son, and with what will you suggest they play? Will she be bringing anything from home or will you use what you have?

You can see that careful planning, time to gather what you need, and creative and flexible thinking are essential elements of the therapy process.

Outcomes/criteria for success and methods of recording

The question to ask of yourself and your client is 'Have the objectives been met?' However, other questions will follow this: 'How much help or cueing was needed?' 'What length of time was there before a response occurred?' 'What precision accompanied the activity?' So, if you are to have a clear idea of the usefulness of the therapy session, you need to specify at the outset what level of achievement is to be expected. If the main focus at this time in therapy is a change in attitude or feeling on the part of the client, it is less easy to be specific but still possible to consider some rating or measure of attitude change.

You can use a framework such as the one in Figure 4.5 to help you decide how to specify outcomes.

As an example of the recording and measuring of objectives, we can again look at the plan for George. The objective that George will gain attention four times should be easily measured as long as there is an appropriate way of recording every time he makes an attention-getting action. If you do not have at the very least a notebook in which to write down these attempts you will be left at the end of a session (in which numerous events have occurred) trying to recall whether it was four or three or maybe five times that George moved his paper, pointed, and so on.

The second objective set for George – that he should produce an initiation of conversation in some way – is more difficult to measure. What criteria can you and he set that will be observable? Will he be expected to initiate quickly, slowly, with help, with no help? You may both decide that at this point in time he will need some support to make an initiation but that, before the help from you, George will be given some time to generate an idea. You could produce a chart together such as the one in Table 4.1.

A record such as this will prove invaluable in the final process of the session plan – the evaluation.

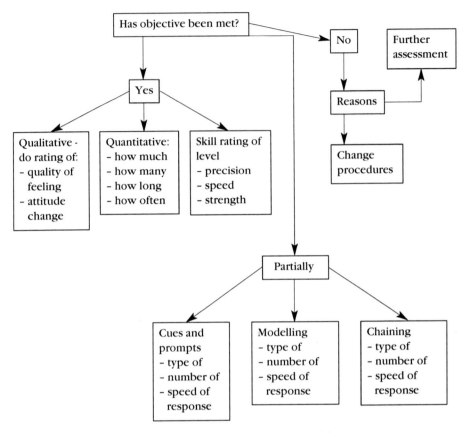

Figure 4.5 A flowchart to guide consideration of outcomes of therapy.

Table 4.1 A record chart for measuring outcomes

Attempts	Spontaneous (quick or slow)	Non-verbal prompt (nod or gesture)	Verbal prompt (non-specific, e.g. yes?)	Verbal prompt (direct, e.g. was it about 'x'?)
1				
2				
3				
4				
Comments				

Evaluation of session

To evaluate the session successfully you need to ask yourself the following:

- Did the session meet its objectives?
- If so, how and why?
- Where do we go from here?
- If it did not meet its objectives, why not?
- What is needed to improve the outcomes?
- What was the client's experience?
- What part did I play in the process?
- Was the overall timing about right?

Criteria for discharge (leaving)

Decisions about terminating therapy will be based on the original long-term aims and the change that the client has undergone since entering the therapy process. (Bunning [2004] discusses Pound et al.'s [2000] use of the word 'leaving' instead of discharge as an active choice made by the client rather than a clinician-initiated decision.) Regular evaluation of sessions in the light of movement towards final outcomes will be needed. These evaluations should be joint ones and will be based on some form of measure of change. Termination of therapy may occur as a result of a number of factors:

- Satisfactory achievement of long-term aims.
- Mutually agreed discharge before aims are met.
- Other agencies taking over the client management, e.g. the special needs team in a school or the community team for adults with learning difficulties, etc.
- Referral to another professional or to another speech and language clinician for a different therapy approach.

Therapy outcome measures have been the focus of much discussion and work over the past few years. Because people and language difficulties are very complex and, because change can take place at a number of different levels, it is difficult to give a simple answer to the question 'Has your client improved, and by how much?' Discussion in 1997 (Rossiter 1997) in the Royal College of Speech and Language Therapists' (RCSLT's) bulletin took up the issue of outcome measures and warned against trying to be too global, i.e. covering everything possible in one measure. Rossiter (1997) showed that measures such as a Functional Independence Measure are invalid in terms of identifying change over time. A good critique of some of the measures used is provided by Hickman (2002), who identifies the problems of subjectivity and reliability that occur in many general measures. However, it is essential that a speech and language clinician find some way of measuring clinical effectiveness. There is a growing awareness that measures must take into account the client's own thoughts about his process of change. In the fields of stammering and voice therapy, client rating scales have become an essential part of decision-making about outcomes. An example of this is to be seen in a scale such as the Wright and Ayre Stuttering Severity Profile (WASSP – Wright and Ayre 1998).

However, you must consider a number of different ways of measurement, including rating scales. These may be through a range of different methods such as:

- re-testing of previously tested areas
- further recordings and transcriptions of these to identify change
- use of a number of charts and rating scales
- client satisfaction measures
- satisfaction of involved others
- reported change by others in language, or school behaviour, etc.

Discharge or leaving is not seen as absolutely final. In many services, discharge is a part of the process of turnover of caseloads and many clients may appear again at a later stage on the referral list. Thus a child aged 4 with language delay may be discharged when language comprehension and language expression are on a par, despite the fact that he or she is still testing out as below norms. This child may be re-referred at age 7 by education because of continuing phonological delay that is impacting on literacy (Bernhart and Major 2004). Another example may be an adult who stammers, is discharged and joins a self-help group where his ability to control his stammering is maintained to a reasonable extent. However, a year later he may apply for a new job and may wish to revise some of the techniques that he has learned so he approaches the service for additional therapy sessions.

The therapist in therapy

We have talked about therapy as being an agent of change in the client. But it also changes the therapist. You cannot engage in a therapeutic relationship with a client without this influencing you. You need to be self-aware and self-evaluating in order to make use of these changes in yourself and to grow and develop as a professional. Reflective practice is a cornerstone of current thinking in education and health. Based on the seminal work of Schön (1987) professionals are encouraged to reflect on action (the things you did in therapy), feelings (the way in which you managed the process emotionally) and learning (what came out of the process that taught you something new). Self-examination can feel threatening to start with. During your university education you will have been encouraged to start this process, but remember it is a lifelong one, you cannot put it aside as you enter your profession. Bannister (1982, p. 202) points out:

To try and understand oneself is not simply an interesting pastime, it is a necessity of life. In order to plan . . . and to make choices, we have to be able to anticipate our behaviour in future situations. This makes self-knowledge a practical guide, not a self-indulgence.

You regularly need to consider the following:

- What sort of a person you are – your underlying philosophy of life
- What your strengths and weaknesses are
- What needs you are fulfilling in therapy. Maslow (1968, in Leahy 1995) suggests that there is a hierarchy of needs for all human beings, of which the need for love and belongingness, that for esteem and that of self-fulfilment would be potentially met for the therapist in a therapy relationship
- What beliefs and attitudes bias or guide your therapy
- Which personal relationships are potentially likely to intrude into the therapy situation
- What, from your past life, may be influencing the way you feel about this client.

And more – the list could go on. And why is it done? Green (1992) puts forward reasons why regular reflection about work is important:

- To help therapists deal with issues relating to their involvement with clients and with the personal and professional difficulties that can arise from this.
- To protect the interests of clients and ensure that therapists are supported to do this.
- To offer support to therapists and detect early signs of difficulties.
- To challenge therapists on their work practices in a supportive, trusting environment.

Supervision is encouraged in speech and language therapy. This is a process that enables you to discuss your work and your feelings about your work regularly with someone who is experienced and qualified (RCSLT 1996). It is an essential part of being a reflective practitioner.

We have now considered what therapy is, the framework on which you might construct your therapy, the way in which you go about planning your sessions, and the processes that you go through as you develop your role as a speech and language clinician. Your primary aim must be to provide a facilitative context in which your clients can change in a positive direction.

Using the process – therapy plans

Below are four different plans based around different clients with different needs. These have been chosen to provide examples of how planning, while maintaining the same systematic and careful structure, can have different content related to the philosophy behind the approaches and the context and situational demands made.

The first plan considers a pre-school child with specific ethnic and gender issues in a child development centre; the second takes a child of primary school age and looks at planning within the educational setting; the third considers an adult client with aphasia and the issues of planning to meet his psychosocial needs; and finally a group plan is presented focusing on social communication skills with clients with learning difficulty.

Case discussion: client 1 – Asha

Asha was referred with her family to the child development centre by a health visitor when she was 2;06 years old. There were general concerns about her language, her play and her overall development. Asha had 'unusual' tics and movements, and she screamed a great deal which was obviously causing the family distress. She was the seventh girl in a culture that valued males. There were obvious frictions caused by this, and her father showed little interest in her welfare. Her mother, however, was very anxious about Asha's development and showed a willingness to comply with therapy.

World Health Organization (WHO 2001) classification of Asha's presenting difficulties

- **Impairment**: delayed language and play.
- **Activity limitation**: inability to play with friends/family; inability to occupy herself; lack of ability to make her needs successfully known; lack of opportunity to communicate as family 'speak' for her.
- **Participation restrictions**: family rarely take her out because of concern about reactions of others; child not involved in family activities, events; treated as baby by siblings.
- **Distress**: father feels the need to reject her because of gender and slowness of development; mother anxious about development; whole family upset by screaming; possibly screaming is related to child's frustration.

Client 2 – James

James was brought to the attention of the speech and language therapist by his class teacher. James had received therapy when he was 3 and 4 years of age. He had had problems of listening and attention and slow expressive language development. He was discharged with minor phonological delay. James was now in school and was having difficulty with the demands of Key Stage 1 of the National Curriculum (Department for Education and Skills 2004). At 6 years of age he was the second child in a busy family. His parents were concerned about his difficulties at school and often compared his progress to that of his 8-year-old sister who was doing extremely well.

WHO classification of James's problems

- **Impairment**: delayed expressive language development; phonological delay.
- **Activity limitation**: difficulty with listening in school; reading and writing slow; access to the curriculum is reduced.
- **Participation restriction**: possible peer group attachment difficulties linked to activity limitations.
- **Distress**: parents anxious; comparisons with sister may cause sibling friction; child may become aware of problems and react negatively.

Client 3 – Harry

Harry was a successful businessman when he had a stroke age 56 years. The stroke left him with a weakness on his right side, which limited his mobility and restricted activities such as driving, golf and gardening. The stroke also left him with reduced ability to follow conversations (especially in noisy or distracting environments), significant problems with word-finding, a slowness in his reading that leads to problems of recalling what has been read, and problems in the area of writing. He was unable to continue in his job and he found his restricted daily activity very disturbing. His wife had to increase the hours that she worked and Harry disliked his financial and emotional dependence on her.

WHO classification of Harry's situation

- **Impairment**: receptive and expressive aphasia, some reduced mobility.
- **Activity limitation**: difficulty expressing thoughts and ideas to others; inability to read for pleasure; reduced ability to contribute to group conversations; loss of work; loss of independence related to lack of driving; loss of access to leisure activities (golf).
- **Participation** restriction: reduced financial security; reduced meeting of other people, loss of friendships; changed and diminished role and responsibility; loss of self as active organizer of other people.
- **Distress**: anger and withdrawal; anxiety of part of wife; fear of the future.

Client 4 – Sam, Frank, Malik, Lucy and Ayshea

Sam, Frank, Malik, Lucy and Ayshea all attended a local college of further education where they were involved in different programmes aimed at developing their life skills and independence. All of these young people had had problems of learning and managing their daily lives from birth. However, each had individual strengths that were tapped in the social communication group that they attended. Sam had Down's syndrome and came from a family who had always seen him as just another family member, not a person with problems. He was well travelled and had a wonderful photograph album of the countries he had visited. Frank and Malik had epilepsy, which had restricted their lives to some extent. Frank was a joker and made friends easily whereas Malik was quiet but sensible and kept the group in order if things got noisy. Lucy, who had cerebral palsy, was the oldest member of the group and often took the 'mother' role, especially if someone was upset. Ayshea was the youngest member. She loved the games and activities and was quick to volunteer and be involved. She had fragile X syndrome.

WHO classification for the different group members

- **Impairment**: all group members had receptive and expressive language difficulties. They also had cognitive problems that resulted in some pragmatic difficulties.
- **Activity limitation**: for all members of the group, getting their ideas across to those who did not know them well was a major problem; access to community events and reduced independence linked to these problems; initiating contact with others was reduced for Malik and Lucy.
- **Participation restriction**: making and keeping friends and sharing ideas about themselves was reduced; fulfilling an adult role in society was a hope for Frank, Malik and Lucy but this was difficult given the restrictions above.
- **Distress**: Lucy became upset when she was rebuffed by others; Malik could easily withdraw if not understood; Frank showed some anger when people whom he thought were his friends rejected him; Ayshea and Sam's parents were concerned about the long-term situation for their 'children'.

Philosophy of treatment

Each of these clients presents with a unique set of issues that the speech and language clinician must take into account. Within each setting certain philosophies and ideas hold sway. The therapist must work within these as well as bring her own beliefs and self-knowledge to the planning and active undertaking of therapy.

Asha must be considered in the light of her family's beliefs about her place in their system. How is her gender and her disability seen by the immediate and the extended family? What effect will the family belief system have on the process of her therapy? The child development centre adopts a family systems approach (Barker 1998) and believes that treatment of one member of the family in isolation is inefficient and inappropriate and that as many of the members of the family as possible should be involved. These ideas will influence the plan of management that will be drawn up.

James needs to be able to access the school curriculum. The longer he is left struggling with literacy, the more he is likely to feel different from his peers and the more he will fall behind his classmates. On the whole, schools are driven by a behavioural philosophy (Herbert 1981) where targets are set, tasks are broken down into small steps and pupils are taught through the media of modelling, prompting, chaining and reinforcing. James's family are highly anxious. They need to understand the possible negative impact of too much pressure on James and to embrace a more child-centred, encouraging and sustaining approach to him at home. The speech and language therapist will need to embrace both these philosophies in order to plan James's programme effectively.

Harry has undergone significant loss. The effects of his language and mobility problems on his lifestyle and his sense of self, as well as the impact of his difficulties on others around him, are the major issues that will drive the decisions made about his therapy. Harry and his family are struggling with loss of core constructs (Fransella and Dalton 2000), which are the ways of knowing and thinking about the self and of relating to the world. Sudden changes in their lives have raised questions about how life is to be led and how relationships are to be maintained. The therapist will need to try to understand how Harry is seeing himself now in order to help him change and reconstrue himself over time. Personal construct theories will provide some support.

The group will present the speech and language clinician with a challenge in terms of understanding the significance of each client's difficulties as well as planning to meet individual needs within the group framework. Social communication difficulties can be dealt with only in a socially communicative group (Brumfitt 1999). Understanding how to develop and lead the group will be an essential starting point for the therapist. Consideration, from a social contructionist view (Clegg 1993), of the way in which these clients are struggling to access the community in an often hostile social environment, and finding ways of breaking down externally imposed barriers will be part of his or her role. Giving members of the group the opportunity to be listened to while they talk about themselves and tell their life stories (Gray and Ridden 1999) will be an essential aim of the therapist.

Knowledge

For each of these clients the therapist will need to make sure that his or her knowledge base is secure. A sound knowledge of child development and child psychology (Oates and Grayson 2004) is necessary to understand Asha's developmental delays and her unusual behaviour. Exploration of her difficulties will be broad-based and, in the child development centre, will be multiprofessional. The speech and language therapist will need to be sure of her role and her boundaries within the team as well as accepting the expertise of her colleagues. For James, knowledge of the education system, and particularly of the curriculum, awareness of the service agreements between health and education, and the speech and language therapist's role within this, and understanding of James's linguistic difficulties and their link to literacy (Hesketh 2004) are all essential in the efficient planning of his programme. Knowledge in the area of aphasia will be the foundation of work with Harry. In addition, an understanding of the different levels of therapeutic intervention, at the level of the individual, the social context, the community and/or the wider society (see Byng et al. 2000, for a useful table of goals of intervention at different levels) is essential. Managing group therapy demands a knowledge of how to set up and run groups, the social psychology of group behaviour and the roles of group members. Also, literature on the language, cognitive and affective difficulties experienced by people with learning difficulties is required (Rondal and Edwards 1997).

Therapy is designed to bring about change. How an individual may respond to demands for change and how he or she may react to change as it is occurring is important knowledge for the therapist. Prochaska and DiClemente's model of change (1986), mentioned in Chapter 1, is an excellent discussion of the way in which change is facilitated or prevented by the level of awareness of the individual, group or organization. An understanding of the processes that make change painful can be reached through a study of the 'constructs of transition', which define what happens to an individual when he or she is put under pressure to change or to look at him- or herself differently, i.e. the individual is moving, or in transition, from one state of being to another (Dalton and Dunnet 1992).

Skills

For each of these clients, the assessment and therapy approaches will be different. But what are the similarities? Which skills that the clinician brings can be transferred from one to another?

- Careful gathering and recording of data are needed for each of these clients. No matter how different their presenting language problems, the clinician must be able to record, transcribe and analyse their communication, language and general behaviour.
- Joint working, collaboration and shared problem-solving with the organizations and/or individuals are essential for effective assessment and treatment.
- Thoughtful planning, which may require compromise and negotiation, is needed to act as a blueprint for focusing the assessment or therapeutic endeavour.
- Constant questioning of the data and the decisions made is required. The therapists must engage both alone and in collaboration with involved others in problem-solving, analytical thinking and creative theorizing, leading to hypothesis generation about the problem and the management thereof.

Asha

Assessment

Joint assessment to discover Asha's strengths and areas of difficulty took place in a multidisciplinary team at the child development centre. She attended for a morning with her mother and one of her sisters. The full team at the centre consisted of the consultant paediatrician, occupational therapist, physiotherapist, speech and language therapist, play therapist, clinical psychologist, educational psychologist and health visitor. As Asha had been seen at home by the health visitor, who had identified play, behaviour and language as the main issues, the team on this particular occasion consisted of only three professionals who would hand on their information and ask for additional input from the others should this seem necessary. Asha was taken to the playroom with her mother and sister, where she was free to play while her mother was asked, by the clinical psychologist, about the difficulties at home. Her play was observed by the play therapist and speech and language therapist, and her interaction and attempts at communication with her sister and mother were noted. During this period, the speech and language therapist hypothesized that Asha was seemingly uninterested in engaging others in communication and that this may be linked to the fact that she was not being encouraged to play or interact by either her sister or her mother. The therapist then entered the playroom and tried to engage Asha in play. Asha's response was observed by the play therapist and clinical psychologist. She appeared interested for a short while but when pressured in any way she started crying. Her mother reported that she 'muddled in' with all the others at home and that her problems had not been considered as severe, except for her screaming. After a careful case history and observation, the team met to share their findings and developed the following hypotheses:

- Asha appeared to be slow at development in the areas of fine motor skills, play, language and problem-solving.
- Her screaming behaviour could relate to an inability to achieve her ends in a busy household where she received little individual attention.
- Her mother seemed keen to help but a bit overwhelmed by the family pressures and under-supported by the extended family, which she put down to her inability to have a boy child.
  A management plan was drawn up which consisted of the following.

Aims

- To explore further the nature of Asha's difficulties by home visits and referral to the occupational therapist.
- To ascertain the level of awareness and involvement of members of the family.

- To encourage Asha's mother to consider nursery placement.
- To rule out, if possible, certain diagnostic possibilities such as autism.

Objectives

- That Asha will have been observed in the home, and her play, communicative ability and general behaviour recorded over a longer period.
- That Asha's mother will have been offered support in terms of a nursery placement and possibly some help with Asha in the home if appropriate.
- That Asha's fine motor skills will have been assessed.
- That relationships and support within the home will have been explored through further discussion with Asha's mother and sisters and meeting Asha's father.

James

Assessment

James was seen in school where the speech and language therapist could see him in the classroom and alone, and have discussions with his teacher and the special needs coordinator. Time was constrained by school routines so the therapist arrived at break (she was already known by the school) and spoke briefly to the teacher to ascertain the teacher's level of concern. After break she joined James in the classroom where she was able to observe and record his behaviour in relation to his peers. She participated in the literacy hour where again she was able to identify his level of competence and finally she spent 15 minutes alone with James, during which time she chatted to him and conducted a quick screening of his expressive language using the Renfrew Action Picture Test (Renfrew 2001) which she recorded for phonological analysis. She also completed with him some subsections of the Phonological Assessment Battery (Fredrickson et al. 1997) to see whether James had difficulty with phonological processing. At the end of the day, the speech and language therapist met with the special needs coordinator to report her findings and look at how James could be supported in school and within the everyday curricula activities. After the observations and assessments it was felt that:

- James stopped listening to stories or commands that contained more than four pieces of information – suggesting some difficulties processing longer sequences.
- James's grammar was more delayed than his ability to convey content of pictures (as identified by the Action Picture Test) but both were within normal limits.
- James showed continuing immaturity of phonology (he was still reducing some /s/ clusters) and this might impact on his reading.

- James struggled dealing with rhyme and with understanding that sounds constituted onsets on words – this would affect his reading ability.

A joint programme was set up for James that linked the aims of his speech and language therapy with the curricular aims of the speaking and listening and the reading attainment targets set by the National Curriculum for children at Key Stage 1 and the objectives with the goals of his individual education plan (IEP).

Aims

- To encourage James to listen carefully and respond appropriately to commands.
- To assess further the strategies that James appears to be using in attempting to read texts.

Goals: linked to listening

- James will listen to stories with first three, then four, then five pieces of information.
- James will correctly answer questions related to stories containing three pieces of information.
- James will correctly carry out commands that contain five pieces of information.

Goals: linked to reading

- Class teacher will identify whether James is using phonic and/or graphic and/or contextual meaning cues in his reading.
- James will learn the rules of simple rhyming (an understanding of onsets and rimes in words).

Harry

Assessment

Assessment of the strengths and problems that Harry and his wife bring to the management of their own change took place within the hospital-based clinic room. Careful planning of the seating arrangements was done by the therapist, so that both Harry and his wife would be fully involved in the discussion of their needs. Through conversation, discussion and a selection of comprehension pictures from the Sentence Processing Resource Pack (Marshall et al. 1999), the therapist was able to obtain an overview of the situation in relation to the language difficulties, the ability of Harry and his wife to manage conversations between themselves, the most prominent difficulties that they are facing in adapting to the lifestyle changes, and the emotional state and readiness to change for both of them. The assessment ended with joint consideration of the possible options for management:

- That Harry and his wife might find easier ways to communicate with support.
- That some direct work on strategies for word retrieval and recall of read passages might be of benefit to Harry.
- That support from an organization such as Different Strokes (see www.stroke.org.uk) (which has been developed to help the younger, more active people who have had strokes) might be worth exploring.
- That Harry and his wife might consider some counselling (separately or together) to help them deal with the sudden changes that they have undergone.

It was decided by the couple that they would like to work on supported conversation (Lock et al. 2001) and Harry also wished to try some individual work on his problems of word-finding and reading. They also felt that some time just talking with the therapist about the stroke, the aphasia and the implication for them might be useful. At this point in time they did not wish to explore more formal counselling or the support group, but they were happy to keep this in mind. Consequently, the following aims and objectives were set.

Aims

- To look at ways of changing communication skills used by both Harry and his wife.
- To develop different modes of communication.
- To assess word retrieval and reading difficulties further in order to devise appropriate tasks related to these.
- To explore the anatomy and physiology of stroke and the ways in which language can be affected with the use of diagrams, models and other visual aids.

Objectives

- That Harry and his wife will attend four sessions to explore and practise different ways of communicating and conversing with on another.
- That they will practise communicating in a number of contexts outside the clinic.
- That subtests of the Psycholinguistic Assessment of Language Processing and Ability (PALPA – Kay et al. 1997) and informal assessment of response to cues will be used to explore Harry's word-retrieval difficulties.
- That Harry and his wife will explore at home the range of literature that they would be likely to read and the particular areas of difficulty that Harry is having.

- That two sessions would be set aside early in the course of therapy to explain and discuss the stroke.

At the end of 6 weeks, another planning meeting would be held to decide on future options.

Sam, Frank, Malik, Lucy and Ayshea

Assessment

As all of these young people have probably been known to the speech and language service on and off over a number of years, the therapist would need first to try to find past notes in order to obtain an idea of their developmental paths. Also, the college would have information about how each of them is coping on the programmes undertaken there. The knowledge of how syndromes and neurological impairments may affect people would also be needed as a basis for assessing the group. The therapist would then go to the college to use a quick screening of understanding in order to ensure that the group activities are focused at the correct comprehension level for all. A framework, such as the CASP: Communication Assessment Profile for adults with a mental handicap (Van der Gaag 1988), would be useful both for gathering information from others and to assess language skills directly. The level of ability to gesture or sign or use symbols or electronic aids would need to be known in order to plan the group. However, as therapy and assessment are so intertwined, the group may well start and run effectively, with the therapist identifying strengths and needs during the activities. The ability of the group to gel and function well cannot be assessed beforehand; it will depend on the skill of the therapist and the responses of the members.

After discussion, fact finding and brief meetings, the therapist may have the following thoughts and devise the following aims and objectives:

- The general language and cognitive levels of the members of the group are different but not so divergent as to make the group unworkable.
- All students have the understanding and language comprehension to know what we are doing and to follow simple directions.
- Verbal language, gestures, signs and symbols are used to some extent by all.

Aims

- To create a group that is fun and supportive.
- To encourage the use of a wide variety of modes for expression (with particular emphasis on the use of symbols – Widgit Software 2000).
- To develop confidence in engaging others in interaction.
- To enhance communication skills.

Objectives

- That all members of the group will join in games and activities willingly.
- That some members will volunteer games and activities.
- That all will manage to convey messages successfully through a range of communication modes.
- That eye contact, gesture, smiling and waiting while others have a turn will have increased in those members who need these skills.

The aims and objectives presented here for the four clients can be seen as short term, in that they are achievable within a reasonable timespan. They will be part of a more global view that the therapist will have of the long-term outcomes for these clients. The long-term aims will be affected by the nature of the impairment, the degree of activity limitation, the complexity of the difficulties in participation and the levels of distress of the individuals involved. There will also be service delivery issues including attainment targets that will drive short- and long-term decisions.

Plans and outcomes

For two of the clients, an example of how the short-term aims and objectives are converted into a session plan are presented. Harry and the group have been chosen to represent ways of approaching individual and group therapy. For Asha and James, the procedures that are undertaken will be jointly decided with the other involved people (the child development centre or CDC team, the teacher and/or special needs coordinator). In the school setting the possibility is that the therapist will not run speech and language therapy sessions because the goals link to school attainment targets. However, she will monitor and support where necessary.

Harry

After the initial sessions where the issues of stroke and aphasia were explored and further assessment completed on both Harry's word-finding and the conversational patterns of the couple, the therapist has the following thoughts:

> Harry and Julie (his wife) seem to have benefited from a more secure knowledge of exactly what has happened to Harry. They both seem more accepting of the level of his difficulties and therefore more ready for actively participating in therapy. While they both still hope that his speech will improve, they are beginning spontaneously to use more gesture with each other. From the video of their conversation it appears that their difficulties lie mostly in the area of repair and turn-taking. It seems a good time to introduce a more formal approach to their conversational skills.

The following plan was made from session 3.

Aims

- To introduce the video and help the couple to look at it objectively.
- To encourage creative exploration of ways of communicating.
- To practise some communicative exchanges.

Objectives

By the end of the session Harry and Julie will have:
- been able to look at the video and talked about how they converse
- been able to express thoughts and feelings about the video
- chosen a specific area to work on
- brainstormed a variety of ways to change this particular habit
- practised the chosen options using 10 pictures
- discussed their responses to this
- decided on a brief daily practice activity for home.

Procedures

- Talk about ways we communicate and the amount of information we convey non-verbally as well as discuss what we do to repair our messages and how turn taking is used in conversations.
- Show video clips of themselves, making sure there are examples of good message exchange as well as some areas of difficulty.
- Ask for comments on the tape and pick up on any anxiety and emotional content.
- Brainstorm ways to change one chosen aspect.
- Look at a list of options (pointing, facial expression, gesturing, writing parts of a word, miming, drawing, giving verbal clues, etc.) and choose some to try out.
- Use everyday activity pictures to 'talk' about, taking turns to try different methods of communicating.
- Discuss feelings and possibilities.
- Plan homework.

Methods

- Prepare simple tick chart to go with video so we can all identify the aspects chosen as problematic.
- If Harry or Julie seems anxious, spend time talking about conversations and the amount of non-verbal information that we all exchange.
- If they find it hard to identify conversational breakdowns, choose only one and go over it a number of times.
- Ask them to think of times when they have been abroad and how they manage (focus on non-verbal means).
- If this is emotionally difficult, have some pictures of people on holiday and ask them to discuss.

- Ask for comments on the relevance of this to the piece of video that we have observed.
- Use photographic pictures and all look at them one at a time to start with. Model gesture, writing, etc. (whichever has been chosen) and ask for imitation.
- If easy, ask for spontaneous productions rather than following of model.
- Have suggestions available for homework activities in case Harry and Julie find these difficult to think about.

Criteria for success

As this is an introduction to the idea of changing conversational habits, criteria will link to areas on understanding the process and accepting the possibilities of doing things differently. The criteria set will therefore be:

1. Harry and Julie will have shifted their ratings at least one point on scales of understanding and accepting the difficulties they are having, e.g.:

   I can see on the video when Harry says a word that Julie doesn't understand

   Easily　　　1　　　2　　　3　　　4　　　5　　　Not at all

   I can see that Julie starts talking about something else when she doesn't understand Harry

   Easily　　　1　　　2　　　3　　　4　　　5　　　Not at all

2. Harry and Julie will have expressed motivation to try some new ways of helping them understand the messages to be passed by scoring at least 2 on:
   - offering a lot of ideas for things to do at home
   - agreeing to try out some things that the therapist suggests
   - being unsure of whether they can start to change at home.

Evaluation and outcomes

Evaluating the session can be done on the following basis:

- **Were the objectives met?**
  Yes, all objectives were met for this session. It was difficult emotionally and quite a lot of time was spent on discussing feelings and the need for change.
- **How was the scoring on the criteria for success?**
  (a) It was difficult for Julie in particular to identify what she was doing on the tape – she moved only a short way on the rating scale
  Harry was very good at identification (though beware of him focusing too much on negatives). He shifted along the scale quite a way.
  (b) Both scored 2 on the motivation scale.

- **What have we all learned that we did not know before?**
  We all agreed that Harry can use facial expression very well and that Julie needs to look at him more and pick up clues from his face.
- **Was the session successful for Harry and Julie in terms of what they learned and how they felt?**
  It was partially successful. More time is needed and more observation to become skilled at identification.
  It was quite a painful session but both Harry and Julie said that they had benefited from it.
- **What part did the therapist play in the process?**
  The therapist found the session challenging and feels that she needs to discuss it with a colleague for support and guidance.
  She felt that she was sometimes too inclined to put her own view forward instead of giving time and support for Harry or Julie to do so.
  She was pleased with the way in which she managed the recoding equipment and playback.
- **What ideas can be taken forward to the next session?**
  Continue the practice of identification from tape.
  Plan the record forms for the tape more carefully – make them more specific.
  Possibly give Julie a bit of time on her own with the video for additional practice.

The plans prepared for each session for Harry and Julie will be incremental. Each session fuels the following session. What happens in between therapy will also need to be taken into account at the beginning of each session. Change takes place both inside the therapy space and beyond it. The aim is for Julie and Harry to become their own therapists and, when they can manage without the speech and language clinician, they are ready to leave and to seek further help only if negative change occurs.

Sam, Frank, Malik, Lucy and Ayshea

The group will take place weekly for one term. This fits in well with the education establishment and its curriculum. The group is being run by a speech and language therapist and a support worker from the college, and a number of students are involved. Work as a pair is needed for support and to allow for a variety of ideas. It also ensures that the college's goals for the students are being met. By the fifth session, the group are gelling well and the strengths and difficulties of the individuals are more apparent. The plans each week are guided by the events of the previous week, the interests of the participants, and the ideas and decisions taken by the speech and language therapist and college staff members. So the plan that has developed for session 6 is as follows.

Aims

- To encourage peer support during activities.
- To ensure use of gesture, sign and pointing as appropriate.
- To encourage development and use of communication books/passports (Millar 2003).
- To encourage leadership as appropriate.

Objectives

By the end of the session:
- Sam will have:
  taken his turns appropriately
  allowed Lucy to join in without interrupting her
  remembered to use the signs he knows
  added more information to his communication book.
- Malik will have:
  spoken louder during activities
  made more eye contact
  used his communication book when not understood.
- Frank will have:
  identified when he is speaking too much
  asked another to take their turn
  led one of the activities.
- Lucy will have:
  signed her name and what she wants to do
  taken her turn without prompting
  looked at and pointed to named people
  continued to develop her communication passport.
- Ayshea will have:
  encouraged others to participate
  led a number of activities
  used signing to enable Lucy to follow
  helped to plan the next session.

Procedures and methods

1. Introductions and information from the week:
   - Sit in circle, person A walks over to person B, shakes hands and greets, then sits in person B's chair. Person B greets another and so on (encourage eye contact, speaking loudly enough, use of spoken/signed names, waiting for your turn).
   - Music plays, walk around, when it stops, ask the person nearest you what they have done during the week (ask Frank to control the music).
2. Group map of the college (to tie in with college project on finding your way about):

- In two smaller groups with Frank in charge of one and Ayshea in charge of the other, ask students to identify areas, floors and spaces from college, and draw these onto large pieces of paper (encourage students to help each other, let Lucy choose which group she wants to be in).
- Place maps on wall and ask for volunteers to talk about them (encourage signing for benefit of others).

3. Pass the sign game:
   - Stand in a line; the person at the front chooses a picture and signs what is on it to the next in the line, and so on. The final person comes to the front and selects the picture he or she thinks it was (encourage turn-taking, all to use signs, precision in signing, following rules of the activity).

4. Small group work on adding to communication books/passports:
   - Add and discuss pictures taken last week.
   - Put details of Lucy's method of communicating into her passport (give her symbol choices).
   - Ayshea and Frank will discuss activities for next week.

5. Guess who activity:
   - Using chart from previous week of the physical characteristics of each member, prepare symbols to represent hair, eyes, height, other features. One person leaves the room and a group member is chosen.
   - The person from outside returns and has to ask questions to find out who has been selected. Use symbols if needed (encourage pointing, louder talking, fuller questions as appropriate).

6. Break and discussion of additional activities (encourage Ayshea to suggest some activities that she likes, ask for volunteers to lead these).

7. Chosen activity with leader from group.

8. Goodbye activity:
   - Stand in circle, one person calls out something (e.g. people with black shoes) and those who have black shoes go into the centre (encourage listening, awareness, participation, leadership).
   - Finally, call out people who are members of this group – all should go into centre, then all shout goodbye.

Criteria for success

It is not always easy to identify measurable criteria for a group. However, it should be possible to specify how much and how independently certain activities are undertaken by individuals. This would be based on their individual objectives. Charts can be produced that identify specific objectives and each individual can be rated as appropriate (e.g. Table 4.2).

As each activity was carefully matched to the objectives for the clients, it should be relatively easy to answer questions about whether the objectives were met, by whom and how easily.

Table 4.2 Chart to monitor turn taking

Dates	October	November	December
Sam	2	1	1
Frank	1	1	1
Malik	2	2	1
Lucy	3	2	2
Ayshea	1	1	1

1 = no difficulty, 2 = with reminder, 3 = additional prompts, 4 = with full support, 5 = unable/unwilling.

Success in a group is also dependent on how the whole session ran – its timekeeping, the balance of its activities, the amount of interest and involvement throughout, and the pace and flow of the entire session.

Outcomes over 10 weeks

For the group we can look at how the overall programme – the 10 teaching weeks of the term – met its aims and objectives. Each individual's achievements will be considered against the overall objectives.

1. **That all members of the group will join in games and activities willingly**: Ayshea and Frank started with no difficulties in this area. Sam moved from needing prompts to joining in spontaneously. Malik shifted in his ratings from being in need of full support to joining in with occasional encouragement. Lucy showed less change. However, by the end of the 10 weeks she was needing less support (rated at 3 instead of 5).
2. **That some members will volunteer games and activities**: this objective applied only to Frank and Ayshea originally, but it was encouraging to note that Malik began to ask for certain activities. Ayshea moved to a situation of offering suggestions each week. Ratings showed:
   Ayshea: from 3 to 1
   Frank: from 4 to 2
   Malik: from 5 to 4
3. **That all will manage to convey messages successfully through a range of communication modes**: this objective required information from college and home in order for its level of success to be identified. Each student had a profile of skills at college and it was against these that the outcomes of the group were judged. The speech and language therapist also sent home an evaluation form with each student for the family to complete should they wish. Outcomes from these were coordinated to arrive at the data in Table 4.3.

Table 4.3 Chart to show change in ability to convey messages

Name	Conveys a few messages	Conveys moderate number	Predominantly successful
Sam	///////////////////////////	+++++++++++++++	
Frank	////////////////////////	////////////////////////	////////
Malik	/////////////// ++++++	+++++++	
Lucy	//////// +++++++++		
Ayshea	////////////////////////	////////////////////////	//// +++++++++++

Before group: //////. At end of group: ++++++.

4. **That eye contact, gesture, smiling and waiting while others have a turn will have increased in those members who need these skills**: these specific social skills were fairly easily measurable during the sessions. The generalization of such skills is always a problem because they are so dependent on pragmatic knowledge and emotional well-being. At the end of the group it was easy to see that all members were more confident, took turns more appropriately, used eye contact and gesture when engaging others, and so on. Again, it was feedback from others that was needed to identify longer-term improvements in these areas. What could be said was:

• *Activity limitation*: for all members of the group, going out into the community and using the signs, communication books and communication passports that they had developed was the next step. Some change had been noted with Malik and Frank, who had been seen to offer their books to others.

• *Participation restriction*: making and keeping friends and sharing ideas about themselves were seen to change in the sessions. Ayshea's family reported that she was initiating conversations with members of the extended family more. Sam was joining in better when attending a social group.

• *Distress*: Lucy and Malik seemed generally more at ease and were less likely to withdraw if not understood. Sam's and Ayshea's parents conveyed through the evaluation form the information that they felt the communication books had given all the family a better idea of how to move forward with constructing and developing such aids to conversation.

Conclusions

Was the therapy effective? The therapy offered to both Harry and his wife and the group could be seen as having positive outcomes. It is difficult in the short term to draw conclusions about the effectiveness of therapy because effectiveness is linked to permanent change. Many speech and language therapists do not have contact with their clients for long enough to be able to assess such change. This is a problem in being able to meet the challenge of proof of effectiveness so necessary in clinical governance.

However, it is possible to show, given therapy outcome measures, that some positive change has occurred for both sets of clients. Use was made of evidence from outside the clinic and from people not immediately involved in the therapeutic process. This increased the reliability of the evidence and enhanced the acceptability of the conclusions.

General conclusions

The information presented on these three clients will hopefully have made explicit some of the important issues originally raised about the reality of being a therapist. The therapist with each client was operating from a particular philosophical base. The underlying theories touched on were drawn from:

- client-centred therapy
- personal construct therapy
- family/systems theory
- social constructionism
- narrative therapy
- cognitive therapy
- learning theory.

The more aware the therapist is of the different perspectives that can be taken, the more responsive to client needs he or she can be. Overall, the therapist was operating from a humanistic perspective, believing that the client was capable of being able in some way to direct his or her life choices.

The knowledge that the therapist called on actually to conduct the sessions was based on an understanding of:

- language acquisition and development
- bilingualism and language development and use
- phonological processing
- cognitive difficulties (particularly attention and memory) and their links to language
- social skills and pragmatic aspects of language
- augmentative and alternative means of communication.

The therapist found the model of change suggested by Prochaska and

DiClemente (1986) to be invaluable in helping her to make decisions about:
- where to start – at what stage of change is this individual (pre-contemplative, contemplative, active, maintaining)
- where to focus in therapy – what level is most appropriate (symptomatic, interpersonal, systems, intrapersonal)
- what processes are likely to change and what techniques might encourage this to occur (self re-evaluation, environmental re-evaluation, counterconditioning, stimulus control, environmental control, etc.).

The ideas that the therapist came up with, as well as the ways of bringing the changes about, grew out of her knowledge and experience, and her willingness to talk to others and read around the issues. She was able to think creatively because she was secure that she was as knowledgeable as possible, that she could call upon others, that the clients were also involved in the decision-making about their therapy, and that she and her clients were approaching the therapeutic situation with a hypothesis-generating and testing model. She was therefore confident that she understood both the process and the practical aspects of therapy.

Chapter 5
Enabling, collaborating and educating

Chapters 3 and 4 have examined the assessment and therapy process, and focused on relationships with the client. However, most clinical relationships will involve working with a range of other people. The first part of this chapter therefore looks at:

- relationships with families and informal carers
- relationships with professionals
- inter-agency collaboration.

The second section looks at wider aspects of the clinician's role. Although direct intervention with the client, on either an individual or a group basis, may be central to the work, increasingly speech and language clinicians are becoming involved with a range of indirect approaches, including:

- education and training for carers and other workers
- consultancy
- health promotion and policy development.

Working with relatives and informal carers

The relatives or people providing day-to-day care for the client are extremely important. They are likely to have the most amount of contact with clients, and will shape and influence the environment in which communication takes place. Relatives are therefore a great source of support that you can harness in the intervention process. At the same time, relatives and carers may have a high degree of emotional involvement with the client, and may require support and assistance from the professionals involved. For them to provide appropriate support for the client, relatives must understand the nature of the client's difficulties and have realistic expectations for the future. With the client's permission, the clinician may be seeking the perceptions of the problem from the carers, how this impinges on the client's life and what the expectations for change are. It is important that the long- and short-term aims of intervention are negotiated with the client and carers, and meet the client's needs in their particular family and social network.

Consent to treatment

No assessment should begin without prior consent; this should be formally recorded in the client's notes. *The NHS Plan* (Department of Health or DoH 2000a) identified the need to re-form how patients should be asked to consent to treatment, and model forms have been developed (NHS Circular 2001a, 2001b). You should become familiar with your employing authority's own policies and protocols, as well as guidelines provided by the professional body. Issues of confidentiality need to be considered (see Chapter 7) and permission should be gained from the client before sharing information with a third party, even if this is a close relative or co-worker.

Parents and children

The Children Act 1989 reaffirmed the view of the government that children are best looked after within the family and the best way to help the child is by professionals working in partnership with parents. The Act introduced the concept of 'parental responsibility' to replace the previous notion of parental rights. Parental responsibility means that:

- children should not be viewed as the property of parents
- child rearing is primarily the responsibility of parents
- the role of the state is to assist parents with these responsibilities but not to interfere with family life.

It is essential that professionals work in partnership with parents. Every Child Matters Green Paper (Department of Education and Skills or DfES 2003) and the Children Bill 2004 (www.Publications.uk/pa/pabills) pledge to strengthen the support and involvement of parents, and stress that they should be central to the decision-making process. There is an increasing emphasis on the empowerment of parents within a partnership with professionals. For the speech and language clinician working with children, this relationship with parents should be central to intervention. In the community clinic the parent may often be responsible for bringing the child for the appointment, so that regular contact is established, and good working relationships may be easy to foster. During the assessment the parent will be able to provide a wealth of information about the general development of the child. Parents will be able to give more specific information about the development of communication, and the particular problems that their child is encountering. They should also be closely involved in the decision-making process, and aims and objectives for intervention should be negotiated and agreed with them and with the child, where this is possible. Parents will often be the main implementers of the intervention programme and should, wherever possible, be an integral part of any therapy session. However, the current social context means that many other adults may be involved in the care of the young child, e.g. grandparents, child minders and nursery staff. It will be important to plan with parents how intervention can best be implemented, and who will take responsibility for following it through.

When the speech and language clinician makes recommendations for carry-over work to be continued at home, it is important that realistic and achievable demands be made on the parents. Suggestions need to take into account the home environment, the understanding and capabilities of the parents, and the other demands made on their time from work and family life.

It is extremely valuable for you to observe and work with the child in the home environment. This allows you to:

- observe the child's communication skills in a naturalistic setting
- assess the demands made for communication within the home
- formulate an intervention plan that capitalizes on the environment, utilizes the resources of the home and fits into the family routine
- make a more realistic assessment of what can be expected in terms of home support
- encourage the parents to express their opinions in a familiar environment, where they may feel more confident and in control than in the clinic setting
- encourage the child and the family to see the intervention as part of the everyday context, thereby encouraging generalization and carry over.

There are an increasing number of intervention programmes that have been developed to involve and empower parents in the management of the child's communication problems, e.g. the Hanen approach consists of a series of training sessions for groups of parents (Girolametto 1988). Here parents are encouraged to share their experiences with others in a similar position. The programme aims to influence their attitude to the child's difficulties, as well as teaching them skills to facilitate language development.

For clinicians working in schools, this continued and active involvement of parents may be more difficult to foster, but is equally important. Parents' consent to treatment must always be obtained before an initial consultation and they should be involved in the initial assessment. They should also receive copies of all letters and reports written about their child. However, after the initial assessment, you as clinician may not have regular contact with parents, and may be working through teaching staff and assistants. However, it is still important that parents are kept informed of what is happening with their children, and that they continue to be involved in the intervention process. Contact may be maintained by:

- inviting parents into the speech and language session
- writing in the home–school diary (these are commonly used in special

schools where children are transported to school by the education authority, so that parents may have little day-to-day contact with the school)
- arranging to see parents when they drop the child at school or collect him or her at the end of the day
- being involved in parent evenings and other school activities
- arranging training sessions, coffee mornings, etc., for groups of parents
- regular contact by phone
- visiting the child at home in the school holidays
- writing regular reports in accessible language
- attendance at annual review meetings.

Children with disabilities

For the parents of children with significant and long-term difficulties there will inevitably be a period of anxiety and confusion as they come to terms with the situation. In the early stages they may experience a range of emotional and practical problems including:

- grieving for the 'loss' of the normal child that they were expecting
- anxiety about short-term health issues
- embarrassment and anxiety about telling family and friends
- readjustment of plans to return to work, arrangements for child care, etc.
- concern about the child's long-term future
- confusion and lack of knowledge about the impact of the diagnosis and the long-term implications in terms of development, education, etc.

It is important that all professionals involved with the child and family be aware of how parents are feeling, and provide appropriate and timely support. Confusion and anxiety can be caused when parents receive conflicting information from different people. It is important that, as a speech and language clinician, you restrict your discussions to areas of direct relevance to communication and feeding issues. It is also useful to establish contact with the other professionals involved with the child, so that you are aware of what other information the parents are being given. Every Child Matters (DfES 2003) advocates the development of a common assessment framework to reduce the duplication of information-gathering by multiple professionals. This approach commonly involves the appointment of a 'key worker' to coordinate assessment and provide a single point of contact for the family.

It is recognized that stress and anxiety influence how people are able to process information. The same details and conversations may need to be repeated several times to parents for understanding to take place and for the information to be assimilated

It may also be useful to put parents in contact with suitable support groups, e.g. the Down's Syndrome Association, Scope, etc. Information about local groups should be readily available. For less common disorders, In Touch and Contact-a-Family can provide invaluable information and aim to put parents in contact with other families experiencing similar difficulties. The internet is also a useful place for information and contacts for parents and professionals. However, there is a danger that parents can become inundated with information from this source, some of which may be anecdotal and conflicting. They may need to be guided by the clinician, to good quality, evidence-based information.

In this discussion we have focused on the parents and primary carers, but it is important to remember that other members of the family will be influenced by the situation. Brothers and sisters, grandparents, aunts and uncles, foster and respite parents, nannies and childminders may all be involved in the care of the child and may be invaluable assistants in the intervention process. They may also need support and information to understand the child's difficulties more fully. However, it is important to remember the issue of confidentiality. Permission must be gained from parents before information is disclosed to other members of the family or other carers involved with the child.

The older child or adolescent

As children move into the teenage years there will be a gradual change in their relationship with their parents. At this time the opinions and influence of their peers will take on greater importance. Young people of 16 are presumed to have the competence to consent to treatment for themselves, and in some circumstances younger children who fully understand the procedure can also give consent (see www.doh.gov.uk/consent for 'Seeking consent: working with children'). It may be the case that the parents are keen for intervention to continue, whereas the child does not see the value. A decision will need to be made as to whose opinion is more important. However, if the child is not interested or is hostile to intervention, the potential for change is likely to be significantly reduced. It may be better therefore for you to discontinue intervention until such a time as the child seeks help for him- or herself. Coming to terms with this decision can be difficult for parents and they may require support from you or from involvement in a parent group.

Child protection

The Area Child Protection Committee (ACPC) will consist of a multidisciplinary team involving health, education, the police and the National Society for the Prevention of Cruelty to Children (NSPCC). The Social Services department will usually be the lead agency and will take responsibility for the service and for maintenance of the Child Protection Register (CPR). It is important that all speech and language clinicians working with children attend local training in child protection so that they are familiar with policies and procedures. This includes how to gain information about children on the

CPR, as well as the procedures to follow if abuse or neglect is alleged or suspected.

The speech and language clinician should be aware of general or specific communication behaviours that could be indicative of abuse or neglect. It is important that this information be clearly documented, and the clinician prepared to give evidence in court (see Chapter 7). The Victoria Climbié Inquiry highlighted the failure of professionals to collect basic information and share it across agencies. Every Child Matters (DfES 2003) advocates the development of an information hub in each area to ensure that information is shared effectively. It also suggests the introduction of a common assessment framework to ensure that information is collected effectively and efficiently.

The adult client

With the older child or adult client there may be little or no involvement with other members of the family. Any discussion with a third party must be only with the permission of the client. However, the involvement of family and friends can be an extremely useful part of the assessment and intervention process. It can provide a view of the client's day-to-day communication difficulties, and his or her current lifestyle and communication needs and frustrations.

Before the clinician examines, treats or provides care for a competent adult she must obtain consent (NHS Circular 2001a). It is commonly believed that a parent can continue to give consent for their grown-up child if it is felt that he or she is unable to give consent, e.g. because of a severe learning disability. However, no one can give consent on behalf of an 'incompetent' adult, although treatment can be provided if it is felt to be in his or her best interest. This decision should be made in consultation with all those who are close to the individual. The Mental Capacity Act 2005 will further clarify and strengthen these rights and provides a code of practice for professionals. This will also include guidelines for assessing a person's capacity to consent.

Adults with an acquired disorder

For you to gain information about clients with acquired communication difficulties, relatives and friends may need to be available to provide examples of levels of communication in the home and lifestyle before the trauma. They will also be able to discuss the demands currently being made on the client and the present communication needs.

Case

Mrs S is 85 years old, lives alone and has recently had a stroke resulting in severe mixed aphasia. You learn from her daughter that, before her stroke, Mrs S spent much of her day reading books provided by the mobile library. She was unable to get out to the shops so she provided her daughter with a weekly list of requirements. This information will influence the priority that needs to be given to reading and writing skills, or providing alternative ways to support this activity.

It should also be remembered that relatives are likely to be going through a period of readjustment as they came to terms with the changes that have occurred in their loved one. The communication problem may mean that the client can no longer be as involved in family discussions and decision-making. Both they and members of the family may need support to adjust to these changes in role.

Relatives and friends may also be a useful therapeutic agent and should, wherever possible, be involved in the intervention process. They may want to attend all therapy sessions or visit intermittently, or contact may be maintained through telephone or letter. However, all contact and discussion must be with the consent of the client. In some cases, clients may not wish to have their relatives involved. In other instances, the relatives may not want to attend clinic sessions. The time that the client spends with you may give family members a brief respite from the demands of caring for the client. There may also be times when relatives may wish to talk to the clinician without the client being present. This may give them an opportunity to express feelings and ask questions that they would not do in front of the client.

This support to relatives should be an integral part of the intervention process. It should help them to come to terms with what has happened, and to understand the impact on the client's ability to communicate. It should also provide strategies to help them communicate effectively with the client. It may also be helpful for you to arrange for relatives and friends to meet others in a similar position so that they can share experiences and discuss different ways of handling the situation.

Adults with a non-acquired disorder

For adults who have had a life-long communication difficulty, e.g. a developmental learning disability, there may be a period of adjustment as parents come to accept that their child is becoming an adult. There is likely to be a number of changes in roles and relationships, with the 'child' taking greater responsibility in the decision-making process. At this time, there may also be changes in the communication expectations and demands made on them. These periods of transition from school to work and from family home to independent or sheltered accommodation can mean that existing communication abilities may be challenged. Families may have a well-established routine of communication where they have 'tuned into' the client's system. There may be a need to extend communication skills or provide some sort of augmentative system to facilitate communication with a broader range of people.

Vulnerable adults

These individuals can be extremely vulnerable, and it is known that they are at increased risk of physical, emotional and sexual abuse, and neglect. *No*

Secrets (DoH 2000b) provides guidelines for the development of multi-agency policies and procedures to protect vulnerable adults from abuse. This is particularly important for clients who have severe communication difficulties and may be particularly at risk; they may need sensitive support to voice their concerns. Most areas will have an advocacy service that may be able to provide independent support in these situations.

Working with and through other staff: professional relationships

When you are working as a speech and language clinician, collaboration will be an essential professional skill. You may collaborate with individual colleagues employed by the same organization or those from other public sector agencies, such as education or Social Services departments, or the private and voluntary sector. Partnership working and joint initiatives mean that you may find yourself working in a range of multi-agency settings. This collaborative approach can significantly enhance the client's experience. However, you need to be aware of different professional and employment guidelines and policies, and varying attitudes to confidentiality and record-keeping among staff employed by different agencies.

Case

A speech and language clinician is seconded to a social services project to provide intensive support to children with challenging behaviour. She is employed by her local primary care trust and works alongside a teacher (employed by education) and a care manager (employed by social services). They each have policies, protocols and guidelines laid down by their employing authority!

The list of other professionals involved with the client is not exhaustive, but examples might include the following:

- Health:
    - physiotherapists
    - nurses
    - health visitors
    - health-care assistants
    - consultants
    - GPs
    - clinical psychologists.
- Education:
    - portage workers
    - staff in early years settings
    - teachers

- teaching assistants
- educational psychologists.
- Social welfare:
  - social workers
  - residential and day-centre support staff
  - care assistants
  - occupational therapists.
- Voluntary sector:
  - staff and volunteers engaged by specific service user or support groups, e.g. the Stroke Association, Invalid Children's Aid Nationwide (I-CAN), or the Association for All Speech Impaired Children (AFASIC)
  - individual volunteers.
- Private:
  - staff in nursing homes
  - independent practitioners employed by a public service agency
  - private clinicians.

Team working is essential to good practice, and the speech and language clinician should become a member of the team around the client.

As well as the benefits for clients, there are also advantages for the staff involved. Collaborative practice in the UK has also been endorsed by the formalization and official recognition of a number of teams, e.g.:

- *The child protection team*: a team usually comprising representatives from education, health and social welfare agencies, as well as the police and voluntary agencies. This team is responsible for the coordinated investigation of suspected child abuse, the maintenance of the local CPR, and the development of appropriate policies and procedures dealing with child protection.
- *Learning disability team*: a team frequently based within a Social Services department, providing a multidisciplinary assessment, support and advisory service for people with learning disabilities and their families. This team usually includes a community nurse and social worker, and may involve physiotherapists, occupational therapists, speech and language therapists, and clinical psychologists.
- *Rehabilitation team*: a team usually based in a hospital's rehabilitation unit. It may be led by a rehabilitation consultant, but will include support from a range of therapy services, a psychologist, and nursing and social welfare staff. The aim of the team will be to provide a coordinated package of rehabilitation and support for clients referred to them.

There has also been increasing emphasis on the need for collaborative practice in a range of government guidelines and legislation.

Children's services

The Laming Inquiry into the death of Victoria Climbié highlighted the need for closer collaboration between professionals. The recommendations from this report provided the basis for the changes introduced through the Every Child Matters Green Paper (DfES 2003) and the Children Bill 2004.

Services to people with a learning disability

Valuing People (DoH 2001a) outlined the government vision for service in the twenty-first century. Central to this is the development of effective collaborative working among all agencies and the establishment of partnership boards to ensure coordinated decision-making between organizations.

The National Service Framework for Older People 2003

This aims to ensure person-centred care and integrated commissioning and provision of service and equipment through the introduction of a single assessment process.

At an international level, the World Health Organization's (WHO's) targets for the *Health for All by the Year 2000* (WHO 1979) stressed the importance of a holistic approach to health and disease. This highlights the importance of cross-professional education and training, and the promotion of collaborative practice.

Team working

Terminology

Before examining some of the issues that need to be considered when working in a team setting, it is important to be clear about the terminology used. This is summarized in Table 5.1, but it is useful to consider each of these terms in a little more detail.

Collaboration

Any example of working together could be described as collaboration. In this context, the term is used to describe informal relationships that would not justify the title of 'team'. The speech and language clinician may collaborate with a colleague when they plan a language group together, or collaborate with a health visitor or GP when concerned about the needs of a particular child in their care. Frequently these relationships are short-lived and client- or problem-focused. The skills of clear communication and mutual respect for

Table 5.1: Definitions

Collaboration: to work jointly together

Group: a number of persons located close together, or classed together

Team work: work done by several associates with each doing a part, but all subordinating personal prominence to the efficiency of the whole

Unidisciplinary: working with colleagues from one's own field

Multidisciplinary: a team comprising members of a range of different professionals, which does not necessarily share working practices or common aims.

Interdisciplinary: working with other disciplines in the development of jointly planned objectives/programmes

Trans-disciplinary: committed to teaching, learning and working with others across traditional discipline boundaries; this is likely to involve the transference of information and skills traditionally associated with one discipline to team members from other disciplines

Inter-agency: working with other disciplines employed by agencies different from our own, this can involve interdisciplinary, multidisciplinary or trans-disciplinary collaboration

---

one another's professional expertise and personal opinion are vital, and these informal links, if managed successfully, may lead to more frequent and longer-term professional relationships.

Groups and teamwork

The terms 'group' and 'team' are often used interchangeably. However, there is an important distinction between them. People may be 'grouped' together for a whole range of reasons, but they may not work together in any meaningful or effective way. Often it is hoped that what may start out as a 'group' will develop into an effective team, which will share skills and knowledge for the benefit of other team members and the clients whom they serve. However, the development of an effective team will involve both time and effort. There has been a considerable amount of research into group and team development. The most important factors appear to be:

- group/team development
- roles within the team
- leadership style
- purpose and tasks
- conflict resolution.

Group/team development

It is now commonly accepted that the group goes through a number of recognizable stages from formation to becoming an effective working unit, or team. Tuckman (1965) suggests that there are at least four important stages to group development:

1. **Forming**: at this initial stage, group members are likely to feel unsure and will be concerned with testing out the boundaries of appropriate and expected behaviour. Individuals will need to define their role and contribution within the group, and check that this matches the perceptions of the other group members. At this stage the group members may rely heavily on the group leader for guidance.
2. **Storming**: as group members become more familiar with one another, conflict may arise. Issues of status, prestige and power may need to be resolved. Members may feel a need to assert and clarify their own role and sphere of influence within the group.
3. **Norming**: gradually, as conflicts are resolved and issues of boundaries and attitudes are clarified, the group may be able to compromise and develop a set of shared attitudes and values. At the same time, more clearly defined role expectations, division of labour and established norms of behaviour may emerge.
4. **Performing**: it is only at this stage that the team members can focus on getting on with the tasks in hand. Hopefully, good communication channels have been established and the team has a sense of shared goals and responsibility.

A fifth stage could be added to this process:

5. **Re-forming**: even an effective group may not be continually harmonious. Changes in group membership, the need to meet critical deadlines, external pressures and changes in expectations may lead the group into another period of uncertainty. At this stage it may be necessary for the group to acknowledge the impact of these changes and cycle back through earlier phases of development.

Roles within the team

It is important that the clinician be clear about her own role and contribution in any working relationship. Are members of the team coming together as equals, with equal responsibility for decision-making? Or is it a relationship of manager and subordinate, mentor and apprentice, student and supervisor?

Frequently, we may fail to negotiate and clarify the issues of expectations and responsibility that may lead to misunderstanding, duplication or neglect of important tasks, poor communication and eventual breakdown in relationships. Bower (1987) identified a number of issues that may lead to stress and burnout for advisory special needs teachers. These factors may also be significant for any professional working in an advisory capacity:

- **Role expectation conflict**: stress is generated as a result of a mismatch between a person's own expectation of a role and the expectations that others have of this role, e.g. this may occur in a school setting where the speech and language clinician and the teacher may have different expectations of the role that they each plays in relation to a child with a specific language disorder.
- **Self-role conflict**: stress can be generated when there is a gap between the way people see themselves and the way they are required to behave. Often professionals may have a clear view of how they would like their role to develop. This may be in conflict with the practical implementation in a particular setting.
- **Role isolation**: stress may occur when the individual feels that those occupying other roles, and with whom she has to interact, are psychologically distant. This can be particularly difficult for the clinician who works in a variety of settings, and spends limited time in one location. She may have little contact with other professionals from a similar background. In this situation, the development of supportive relationships can be difficult.
- **Role overload**: stress occurs when there are too many or unrealistic expectations, even when they are clearly defined. This may be a quantitative or a qualitative overload. For the speech and language clinician, it is important to be clear about what *can* be fulfilled, as well as stating what is not possible, so that overload can be avoided. This can be particularly difficult for the clinician working in a number of settings where staff may be unaware of the expectations and demands of other areas of their work.
- **Role inadequacy**: stress may be created if the worker feels that she has insufficient skills or knowledge to fulfil the role adequately. This may be particularly true for the newly qualified clinician who may lack support and confidence. The opportunity to discuss this with a more experienced clinician through a mentoring process will be vital. This may help to identify areas where additional training and professional development may be needed.

Good communication and negotiation may help to avoid some of the pitfalls associated with team working, but it is important to review working relationships regularly so that unnecessary stress is avoided. In any team context, it is worth spending some time discussing the roles and expected contributions of team members. The following checklist may provide a useful starting point:

- What is the overall shared purpose of the team?
- What is each member aiming to do?

- What does this entail?
- Is the team supported by appropriate management to enable them to do this?
- Who is going to take responsibility for each aspect?
- Is there equal responsibility?
- Who takes overall responsibility?
- Is there equal commitment by all team members?

Considerable work on the definition of team roles has been carried out by Belbin (1993). He defines a range of roles that may operate in a group, and provides a useful questionnaire that can help team members to recognize their contribution to the group. This may also help the team to identify gaps in the 'team profile'. Each role brings its own set of strengths and weaknesses, and it is the overall balance and combination of the team that results in success or failure. The clinician may fulfil more than one role within a team, or take on different roles depending on the composition of the group, the task in hand, and how he or she perceives the role within the particular team.

Case

In an annual review meeting in a special school the speech and language clinician may act as the 'specialist' in relation to the needs of a child with a specific language disorder where the rest of the team will look to her specific expert knowledge. However, during the discussion of other aspects of the child's development, where she has only minimal involvement, she may act as 'chair', keeping the group on task with a more objective view of the situation.

Leadership style

Leadership does not necessarily reside in a particular person or position, but may emerge in relation to the demands of the situation. This role may shift from one group member to another depending on the particular task being undertaken, e.g. in a child protection team the head of Social Services may be the leader in the context of a complex case conference. At other times, the child's key worker (who could be any member of the team) may take a leadership role in the coordination of information and the day-to-day decisions affecting the particular child and his or her family.

In some teams there may be an appointed leader, who is given the authority and responsibility to ensure that certain tasks are completed. Frequently the leader will have been appointed to this position by the organization responsible for the team (health trust, education department, etc.), but in some situations this 'authority' may be given by the group itself, in terms of nominating a leader from within their ranks. The leader's key roles are:

- to ensure that the team is clear about overall tasks, and individual roles and contributions within this

- to keep the team on task and focused
- to allow the team to make decisions.

Being a team player

It is useful to consider what leadership qualities are personally viewed as important, and for the group as a whole to recognize the contribution made by different team members.

In many teams, a newly qualified practitioner may not be in a position of leadership, but her positive contribution to the team may be just as important. Therefore, it is also useful to consider how best she can contribute. Some important characteristics of a good team player include:

- the ability to think for yourself
- knowledge of your own strengths and weaknesses
- awareness of extent and limitations of professional expertise
- clear understanding of the task and purpose of the group
- the ability to express your own view clearly and objectively
- respect for the contribution and expertise of other members of the group
- being prepared to negotiate and compromise on some occasions.

Purpose and tasks

Groups come together for a great variety of reasons. The purpose of the team is likely to influence the composition and working practice of the group members. The team may be established on a fairly permanent basis and the members may spend all or most of their work time as a member of the team. This may apply to a child development team, rehabilitation centre team or staff working together in a special school. In other situations, this team may be established on a temporary basis for the life of a particular project, such as planning a training course or designing a department information brochure. At other times, individuals may be involved with the team for only limited periods of their work, e.g. as part of a feeding assessment team. Many speech and language clinicians may in fact work in a range of different teams during their working week. This may necessitate the ability to switch style and role very quickly and requires considerable flexibility, adaptability and assertiveness.

Much of the time and energy of the team are likely to be focused on the specific tasks allocated to them, i.e. the *task-oriented behaviours*, but it is also important to recognize that other issues may emerge during group meetings. Time may need to be focused on *maintenance behaviours* to build and sustain relationships among group members. These may be important in the reduction of tension and resolution of conflict, and to ensure the effective and coordinated contribution of group members. This can be helped by informal contact or 'team-building' exercises, which may not be related to the tasks of the group, but which serve to establish and maintain good working relationships. Also, within the team, members will have their individual needs to be satisfied, such as the desire for recognition and success. These may lead to *self-oriented behaviours*, which may cause unexpected stresses and 'hidden agendas' that emerge and may impede the completion of the task. Again, it may be important to address these issues outside the focus on specific work tasks (Table 5.2).

Table 5.2 Functions within the group

Task-oriented functions
Initiating: new ideas or ways of looking at the situation
Information seeking: asking appropriate questions
Information giving: clear statement of facts and opinions
Opinion seeking: openness to the views of others
Opinion giving: prepared to express our personal views
Clarifying: restating or questioning
Elaborating: expanding on points made by other members of the group
Coordinating: demonstrating relationship between different ideas and information
Orienting: checking on direction of discussion and keeping on task
Testing: checking that you clearly understand what has been said
Summarizing: drawing information together in a clear manner

Maintenance functions
Encouraging: being warm and friendly to other members of the group
Mediating: conciliating differences in opinion
Gatekeeping: helping others to make a contribution
Standard-setting: how groups will operate, rules, choice of tasks, etc.
Following: serving as an audience for other group members
Relieving tension: diverting attention, smoothing over disagreements

Self-oriented functions
Expressing own perspective
Defending professional or personal perspective
Maintaining own position
Gaining reinforcement and support
Preserving own role

Adapted from Jaques (1991).

Dealing with conflict and team breakdown

There will be times where there will be differences of opinion about the best course of action. It is important that this is dealt with in a mature manner and that differences within the group do not become personal. Conflict can often be resolved if the team can refocus on their defined aims, so that individual differences can be set within the context of the overall needs of the client or situation. Clinical and management support and supervision will be vital at these times, and the clinician should ensure that these channels of support are established and maintained.

The multidisciplinary team

Working in a range of team settings means that the speech and language clinician will need to take on a number of different roles and responsibilities. This may call for an understanding of the contributions and different perspectives of a wide variety of other people. This is not always easy, especially as at present unidisciplinary training may foster a 'professional culture' that encourages a competitive rather than a collaborative atmosphere. Frequently professionals may be unaware of their own particular professional culture and background, which influence their working practice, and may have little awareness and understanding of the norms and practices of other professionals with whom they interact. As well as these professional influences, there may also be organizational and agency differences that may further affect these relationships.

Case

A child protection team may have representatives from social, education and health services, as well as the police and voluntary agencies. This team will have representatives from a number of professional groups, as well as different organizational and managerial structures, and procedures.

Collaborative practice is enhanced if professionals take time to consider their own professional perspective and gain an understanding of the personal, professional, organizational and agency influences affecting their colleagues. It may be helpful to consider the following questions, and then use these as a basis for discussion with colleagues from other professional groups:

- What is the overall purpose of your professional group?
- What are your key professional aims, e.g. are they to cure, teach, adapt, etc.?
- What is the core knowledge on which your profession is based?
- Do you use specific vocabulary that may be misunderstood by others?
- How do you view your relationship with your client? For example:
  - patient/doctor
  - pupil/teacher
  - client/consultant
  - facilitator.
- How do you usually relate to other professional groups?
  - receiving referrals
  - referring clients on
  - as a manager
  - collaboratively.

The Royal College of Speech and Language Therapists (RCSLT 2001) has defined the core competencies of the profession, and has looked at the competencies needed within a range of specialist areas. Similar projects are being undertaken by other professional groups in the UK, such as physiotherapy and occupational therapy groups. It is hoped that this will contribute to a greater understanding between professional groups.

The client as the central player in the team

In most of this discussion the client may have been seen as peripheral to the team, but it is obvious that in relation to his or her particular situation he or she is the 'key player' who should, whenever possible, be the prime decision-maker.

As discussed in Chapter 1, the role of the 'patient' has been changing over the past 20 or 30 years. Patients or clients are now considered as customers or consumers of services, rather than in the traditional 'medical model' of care where they have been viewed as passive recipients of services. If we are truly to work in partnership with our clients, we must enable them to voice their opinions and be aware of the professional power that we hold:

> . . . the professional's world view no longer takes precedence over the client's. Nor does the professional have the right to set the terms of the relationship, to prescribe behaviour and to expect compliance. The relationship is now a negotiated one; and the role of the professional is to develop an understanding of his/her client's perceived needs, and to share his/her expert knowledge and skills, in so far as they serve these needs.
>
> Williams (1993, p. 14)

The speech and language team

The speech and language department may consist of the following staff groups:

- speech and language clinicians
- speech and language assistants, associate practitioners and technical officers
- bilingual co-workers
- administrative staff.

Although each group will have different job priorities and backgrounds, the various members will hopefully work together often enough to develop a shared culture.

The speech and language clinician

The opportunity to work with other speech and language clinicians is often a stimulating and rewarding experience. Here, you share the same educational and professional background, resulting in easy understanding of one another's working methods and terminology. As well as the obvious 'two heads are better than one', other advantages might include the following:

- One clinician being able to focus on observing and recording data while the other conducts the activity with the client
- Use of a colleague as a role model of desired behaviour
- Learning from the expertise of a more experienced clinician
- Viewing the client from two different perspectives or specialisms
- Sharing the workload of administration, report writing, etc.
- Providing and receiving feedback on own performance, language levels, etc.
- Observing and experimenting with different approaches
- Ability to focus attention on the needs of both the client and the relative/carer.

As well as working together directly, contact with others in the same profession is extremely important in terms of emotional and professional support. The RCSLT acknowledges that all newly qualified speech and language clinicians should have access to a mentoring system. Regular contact with a more experienced colleague should be timetabled into their programme. Clinical supervision is now recognized as essential at all levels of the profession. This practice has been well established within social work, but has only more recently been recognized as important by other professional groups. Employing authorities should have a policy regarding the mechanism, frequency and recording of supervision (for further discussion, see Chapter 8).

Speech and language assistants, associate practitioners and technicians

Speech and language assistants have been employed in Great Britain for many years. However, this has mostly been on an individual basis to work with clearly defined client groups, e.g. working with stroke groups, in special schools, etc. Speech and language assistants were not required to hold any formal qualification before employment and worked under the direction of a qualified clinician. In the UK, National Occupational Standards have now been defined (Care Sector Consortium 1996) and these have formed the basis of the National and Scottish Vocational Qualifications (S/NVQ) Care Awards at Level 3. This is equivalent to a university entrance level qualification. The RCSLT has established programmes and assessment criteria for this award so that assistants can work towards a recognized qualification.

The speech and language assistant can be a vital member of the team. Over recent years, speech and language therapy assistants (SLTAs) have taken on more responsibility and have become more skilled. Many have now been regraded as technical officers because of their level of skill and the responsibility that they take on. Speech and language departments may have a system to encourage career progression from speech and language assistant to speech and language associate practitioner and then to technical officer.

Although some may have had little or no formal training, assistants may bring a wealth of relevant experience to the role. Others may have qualifications and specific skills that contribute to the overall effectiveness of the team, e.g. sign language qualifications, information technology expertise. *The NHS Plan* (DoH 2000a) and the Modernisation Agency promote the concept of the 'skills escalator' which should provide a mechanism for progression from assistant through to qualified practitioner.

It is important, however, to be clear about what can be expected of staff (Table 5.3), and what they can take responsibility for. This will be negotiated and should be clearly laid out in their job description. The clinician should also be aware of her supervision, management and training responsibility towards them, and must remember that she remains responsible for client care even when she have delegated some aspects of management to the assistant/technician.

Table 5.3 Role of assistants

What assistants do	What assistants don't do
Carry out routine therapy tasks	In-depth assessment
Help with routine administration tasks, e.g. photocopying, etc.	Answer questions put by carers or other professionals
Prepare therapy materials	Work unsupervised
Keep records about therapy undertaken	Write reports

Detailed instructions or programmes may be left, to be carried out by assistants, but it will also be important for them to work alongside clinicians on some occasions. They will also need to understand the overall aims of the programmes of intervention that they are following. They will need feedback on their performance and how they have influenced the behaviour of the clients with whom they are working.

The guidelines in Table 5.4 may help the speech and language clinician to ensure that the assistants (or others working with the client) are confident about what they are doing.

Table 5.4 Teaching therapy procedures

Guidelines for teaching therapy procedures to others

1. Specify desired behaviour and outcome clearly, and explain *why* it is important.
2. Outline procedures and the rationale for its design.
3. Explain sequence of steps involved.
4. Demonstrate the sequence with the client involved.
5. Ask assistant to review/describe the demonstration, reinforce and clarify the procedure.
6. Provide the opportunity for the assistant to demonstrate the procedure on you or another member of staff if appropriate.
7. Observe assistant carrying out the procedure with client, provide feedback and correct *only* critical aspects of the procedure.
8. Review, discuss and revise as necessary, providing written notes to act as prompt. Discuss and agree how progress is going to be monitored and recorded.
9. Encourage assistant to initiate questions and make contact as necessary.
10. Arrange date and time for review and follow-up.

Bilingual co-workers

Bilingual services for clients with speech and language disorders are being established, particularly in areas with large populations of people from black and ethnic minority groups.

Bilingual co-workers will usually be recruited from the local community and are currently employed and trained by the speech and language department. As well as having in-depth knowledge of the community language(s), they may also be able to provide a wealth of knowledge about cultural issues and the local community. RCSLT (1996) guidelines suggest that co-workers may fulfil the following roles, and they have developed a framework for recruitment and training:

- Gathering case history information from the client or carer in his or her home language
- Assessing and observing the client in his or her mother tongue
- Contributing to the differential diagnosis between a primary language disorder and difficulties arising from English as a second language
- Contributing to the management and therapy of clients whose first language is not English
- Interpreting information between the client and the professional
- Offering written information in the client's mother tongue as appropriate
- Advising on culturally appropriate play and clinical materials.

Not all departments will employ such workers, and even those who are able to will not have resources to employ co-workers speaking all the languages used in the local community. If an appropriate co-worker is not available, then try:

- borrowing the services of a co-worker from a neighbouring trust
- using the facilities of other local interpreting services; these are often available through NHS trust or education/social departments
- seeking the advice of a specialist or adviser on bilingualism, or contacting an appropriate special interest group.

The independent practitioner

This term is used to include clinicians working for independent/non-statutory agencies, as well as those in private practice. The newly qualified clinician may be working with a client who is receiving the services of an independent practitioner. It is important that they build up good communication channels and agree who should be the lead clinician. The Association of Speech and Language Therapists in Independent Practice (ASLTIP) is a network for independent practitioners. They have worked with the RCSLT (2003a) to provide useful guidelines to ensure clear accountability and to avoid confusion (see Chapter 6 for further information).

Administrative staff

Secretarial and administrative staff will be central to the smooth running of a speech and language department. They are likely to be the first point of contact for the client and their families – sending out appointments, taking phone enquiries and messages, and receiving clients at the clinic. It is important that such staff have some understanding of the communication problems that these clients may experience, and have good interpersonal skills in order to make clients feel welcome and at ease. Such staff may also be responsible for:

- typing letters and reports
- maintaining client records
- inputting statistical information on to the computer
- maintaining and recording of equipment and resources.

It is vital that they observe issues of client confidentiality and understand the sensitivity of the information that they handle.

The interdisciplinary team

The interdisciplinary and transdisciplinary team

If the clinician is able to be a part of a team for extended periods of time, she may be able to move towards true 'interdisciplinary' work, where there is joint planning and implementation of intervention, e.g. this may occur in a child development centre where various professionals run joint assessment or therapy sessions with each professional's objectives being integrated to form a holistic programme of management (Figure 5.1).

Example: Child with cerebral palsy

**The physiotherapist, speech and language clinician, and occupational thera-
pist may coordinate their management plans so that all individuals working
with the child both inside and outside the centre are aware of the following:**

- which postures and movements to encourage, and why
- which undesirable motor behaviours to discourage, and why
- which positions make it easier for the child to cooperate, move and communicate
- how to communicate with the child, and levels of communicative ability
- how to develop language and expression
- what sensory and perceptual difficulties are present, how material should be
  presented and what sensory and perceptual experiences to encourage
- what equipment is necessary to aid activities and how these should be used
- how to carry or move the child if necessary
- what toys, activities, etc. can be used to motivate the child and how these can be
  adapted to the child's problem.

Figure 5.1 Joint programme for a child with cerebral palsy.

Transdisciplinary working may emerge as professionals work alongside
each other and there is transference of some skills between the professionals
involved, e.g. this may occur in a portage team where one professional will
be appointed to work directly with the child and the family, but may carry
out a variety of educational tasks under the supervision of other professionals
within the team. It will be important for such a team to have developed
mutual trust and respect for each other's expertise. All group members must
be clear about the limitations of their skills and where professional boundaries lie.

Portage

A home-based teaching service for pre-school children with special needs. Portage
home visitors usually visit weekly and work with parents to plan activities so that
their child learns new skills in small steps.

Wilson and Laidler (1990) describe a successful transdisciplinary rehabilitation team. They highlight two significant factors that are central to the team's
success:

1. Respect for individuals' core expertise, knowledge and experience. This
   is seen to be specific to the professional and not shared with other disciplines.
2. The process of skill blending: through sharing of information and
   techniques particular to the individual client, certain skills are transmitted
   to other members of the team (Table 5.5).

Table 5.5 Skill blending

Example: for the child with cerebral palsy considered earlier

Professions involved	Physiotherapy	Occupational therapy	Speech and language therapy
Core skills	Assessment of physical status Positioning and movement	Assessment of daily living skills Wheelchair assessment Switch access	Assessment for and introduction to AAC Considering communication options
Skill blending	Positioning for activities Lifting and carrying	Positioning of equipment Developing independence	Sign language Encouraging communication Turn-taking skills

Inter-agency initiatives: organizational relationships

Many of the considerations discussed in earlier sections apply to the context of inter-agency collaboration. However, because of the involvement of staff from the different employing organizations, relationships and differences of 'cultural' background may be even more complex. Often these initiatives will be set up and formalized at a managerial level.

In many situations, there may be a 'lead' agency that will take overall responsibility for the project. However, working in such a way as to satisfy the needs and priorities of more than one agency can be very demanding. A clear framework of collaboration or 'service level agreement' should be drawn up between service managers to help to define roles and expectations, in order that the group can move forward in an effective manner (Table 5.6).

Sure Start

Sure Start schemes were introduced by the government to improve services to children aged under 4. This scheme brings together staff from all the statutory agencies as well as voluntary groups. The aim is to work with parents and children to promote the physical, intellectual and social development of babies and young children, and thereby break the cycle of disadvantage for the current generation. Having normal speech and language development has been identified as a key indicator and target, so many Sure Start programmes have invested in speech and language expertise. This has resulted in the development of innovative approaches to engage with previously hard-to-reach groups. There are many speech and language clinicians working in this area. They are likely to be involved in preventive work, as well as providing therapy support to some children. The Every Child Matters

Table 5.6 Examples of interagency initiatives

Service level agreement

Purpose and objectives:
• The service being provided by each agency
• Cost of service
• Date of commencement and review/renewal

Scope of work:
• Standards
• Level of expertise

Performance and reporting:
• How to deal with complaints
• How work will be audited

Management structure:
• Managerial accountability
• Professional accountability

Green Paper (DoH 2004) builds on this work with the development of children's centres in disadvantaged areas. These will offer integrated day care, early education, health and parenting services.

Children's trusts

The government hopes that children's services will be integrated within a single organizational structure; it is expected that these children's trusts will be established in most areas by 2006. They will have clear plans covering the key areas identified in the Every Child Matters Green Paper (DoH 2004):

• Being healthy
• Enjoying and achieving
• Staying safe
• Making a positive contribution
• Economic well-being.

Speech and language therapists are seen as key players in the process, and will contribute to success in all these areas.

Intermediate care teams

Intermediate care teams are:

> . . . services which will help to divert admission to an acute care setting through timely therapeutic intervention which aims to divert a physiological crisis or offer recuperative services at or near a person's own home
> Vaughan and Lathlean (1999, p. 23)

These teams usually involve close collaboration of health services, Social Services and voluntary organizations to provide coordinated assessment and rapid response. These teams may contribute to the management of people with mental health problems, children or older people.

All the considerations described above may seem to make the idea of team or multidisciplinary working rather complex and threatening, but, with thought and planning, it can lead to exciting and innovative opportunities. However, the clinician needs to make sure that she is clear about her own role and expectations before she begins. She needs to develop good interpersonal skills so that she can put her own views across in a clear and assertive manner. Teamwork will inevitably require compromise, but when this works well it can lead to enhanced and coordinated client care, innovative solutions and great personal satisfaction.

Working practices

Education and training

Speech and language clinicians have increasingly recognized the value of giving skills to others in order that effective communication support can be provided in a comprehensive and consistent manner.

Providing training to other professionals and co-workers

Purcell et al. (2000) looked at a range of models for delivering training. They concluded that effective communication training had four main elements:

1. It should take place in the workplace and within the daily working context.
2. It should focus on individuals known to the staff.
3. It should involve senior colleagues from the workplace.
4. It should be based on assessment, documentation and evaluation of clients' communication styles.

Kolb (1994) describes the cycle of experiential learning (see Figure 5.1). This can provide a useful model for planning training, which helps to focus training on the needs and concrete experiences of the individual, and the reflective element encourages learners to relate their learning to their work situation.

It is important that all training be carefully planned. It is useful to consult with those involved to ensure that the content is relevant and pitched at the correct level. Clear aims for the course should be defined and negotiated, and these should be agreed with the management involved. Opportunities for reflection should be built into the learning experience, so that participants are encouraged to consider how new knowledge and skills can be integrated into their working practices, and have a positive impact on their interaction with clients. Training should include an evaluation process and needs to be reviewed and revised on a regular basis (Table 5.7).

Table 5.7 Training

Aims of course	These should be clearly defined and made explicit to participants
Learning outcomes	What do you expect the participants to be able to do as a result of the experience?
Target audience	Is this professionals, carers, mixed audience?
Booking	Who will coordinate this process?
Course fees	How will fees be handled?
Minimum/maximum participants	The size of the audience will affect the types of activities that can be included
Venue	This will also influence the activities that can be planned. Is there room for small group work, etc.?
Presentation style	Will this be formal, group work, etc.?
Resources	Are you going to use of video, OHP, multimedia presentation?
Handouts	What will be their content? Who is going to be responsible for ensuring that sufficient copies are available?
Refreshments	Are these to be provided? How and when will they be served?
Admin support	Do you need help with registration, housekeeping arrangements, etc.?
Evaluation feedback	Will this be at the end of the course, or will there be follow-up later?

Consideration also needs to be made about learning and teaching styles. It is recognized that most people have a preferred mode of learning:

- Visual learners learn by looking. They respond well to interactive, visual and colourful data. They like to visualize the information that they are given, draw images and perhaps use mind mapping as a learning tool.
- Auditory learners listen to information presented to them. They will learn more from the verbal instruction than from text.
- Kinaesthetic learners like to make things and learn by 'doing'. They may not be able to concentrate for long periods of time, and will often 'fiddle' with things when they are listening. They require regular breaks in their learning.

A good training session should take the needs of different learners into account, and provide a variety of learning experiences, which should include planning of activities to help participants to reflect and relate their learning to their current knowledge and work/family situation.

Training for families and informal carers

Many of the considerations described above will be important when designing training for families and carers. However, it is important to remember that their interest will be focused on only one individual. They will need the opportunity to discuss how the issues presented can be related to their own particular situation. The training should be linked to the overall aims and objectives of the client's intervention programme.

Consultancy

The speech and language clinician is increasingly required to act in the role of adviser or consultant, with less direct contact with the clients themselves. This has sometimes been driven by pressure on resources and low staffing levels, but it is increasingly recognized as the most effective way to facilitate sustained change and development. Egan (1978) gives a useful definition of consultancy:

> The CONSULTANT influences the TARGET via the efforts of a MEDIATOR.

In this context the mediator may be the teacher, nurse, assistant, parent or volunteer. This approach can help others to develop skills that can be used in the future, rather than focusing on one-off solutions that benefit only one targeted client. Helping others to define, understand and solve a problem in one context may give them skills so that they can come up with solutions when a similar problem occurs in a new context.

The SEN (Special Educational Needs) Toolkit (Department for Education and Science 2001) recognizes that inclusive schools need school staff who are knowledgeable and confident to work with children with special needs, and that this can best be achieved by a collaborative and consultative approach.

The speech and language clinician will remain responsible for the assessment and identification of goals and objectives, but much of the intervention may be carried out by other individuals in the client's environment. This may necessitate the writing of detailed and clear programmes that can be left for others to carry out. Success will rely heavily on the quality of the relationships established with key staff. Regular contact to review and monitor programmes and to provide training and support for staff will be vital. It can be useful to draw up a contract so that everyone is clear about his or her responsibilities.

Public health, health promotion and policy development

Increasingly speech and language clinician are becoming involved in influencing the wider communication and health agenda by contributing to the development of care pathways, risk assessments, multidisciplinary protocols and operational policies. They have a significant role to play in both health promotion and policy development. Acheson (1998, p. 12) defines public health as:

> The art and science of preventing disease, promoting health and prolonging life through the organised efforts of society.

This emphasis on disease prevention and health promotion is to be delivered through local health improvement programmes (HImPs), primary care trusts, and initiatives such as Sure Start and Healthy Living Centres. The government is encouraging services to move away from a focus on disease to a proactive emphasis on health promotion. For the speech and language clinician this might include preventive work with parents through encouraging positive parent child interaction. Examples include:

- Sure Start projects work with parent groups to identify ways to prevent language delay.
- Clinicians introducing dysphagia screening to identify at-risk clients.
- Contribution to policies to ensure that information is presented in an accessible format.

Increasingly speech and language clinicians will find themselves advocating for the needs of their clients, who may be unable to speak up and lobby for themselves. This may include ensuring that their communication needs are considered and incorporated into local and national policies.

Conclusion

The development of team working and the coordinated support of clients can be of significant benefit to the client, the family and the professionals involved. However, team working is not an easy option, and it requires careful consideration, planning and commitment from all professionals and agencies involved. There is also a need for evaluation and audit of new initiatives so that we can become clearer about what the benefits might be. In addition, we need to identify the factors and influences that go towards creating and maintaining an effective team.

However, it must always be remembered that the key player in this team is the client. Clients' needs and wishes must be seen as paramount in the decision-making process. *The NHS Plan* (DoH 2000a) has strengthened the patient's position in the client:professional relationship. This document outlines a number of initiatives to redress the power balance:

- Public patient involvement (PPI): including the setting up of patient fora to structure the development of services
- Copying letters to patients
- Greater patient choice
- Patient advice and liaison services (PALS): to provide information, facilitate immediate solutions and resolve problems for patients.

All these will impact on the speech and language clinician's role, and how she will contribute to the support of clients in the future.

Chapter 6
The work environment

As discussed in Chapter 5, the speech and language clinician will work in a range of different settings and interact and collaborate with staff from a variety of agencies. In the UK, speech and language clinicians are commonly employed within the National Health Service, and these staff may work in a variety of health-care settings. However, other members of the speech and language therapy department may find that most of their contact is with non-health professionals. Speech and language clinicians may also work within one of a range of interagency initiatives such as Sure Start, Partnership Boards and intensive support teams.

The health context

In England, the NHS is managed by the Department of Health and Strategic Health Authorities. These were introduced in 2002 to lead the strategic development of local health services, to performance manage primary care and NHS trusts, and to support them in the delivery of *The NHS Plan* (Department of Health or DoH 2000a).

Primary care trusts (PCTs) organize the delivery of primary health care through general practitioners (GPs) and other community-based staff. They are the lead organizations responsible for:

- assessing health need
- planning and commissioning services
- provision of services
- improving the health of the community.

NHS trusts are responsible for the provision of services commissioned by the PCTs and the development of clinical networks across the NHS community. There are similar arrangements in Wales, Scotland and Northern Ireland, but the structures are slightly different.

168

Speech and language clinicians may be employed directly by the PCT. Their manager may be a clinical coordinator responsible for a number of professional groups. In this case, the manager may not be a speech and language clinician. In small departments there may be only a small number of speech and language clinicians within this team, and they may have little professional contact with others of the same background, as shown in Figure 6.1.

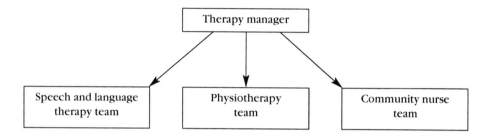

Figure 6.1 PCT-based management structure.

In other areas the speech and language therapy team may be organized as a separate department providing a service across a number of PCTs and community trusts (Figure 6.2). The most likely health-care settings where speech and language clinicians are employed include:

- hospitals
- child development centres
- rehabilitation centres
- community clinics/health centres.

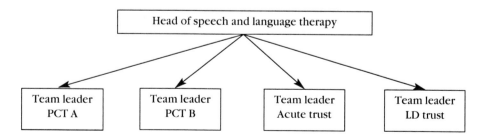

Figure 6.2 Community-based management structure.

District general hospitals and community hospitals

Work here may involve you being in contact with both inpatients and out-patients. Inpatient care may include work on the ward as well as seeing clients who are brought to the department from the ward. It is essential that all other professionals involved with the client are aware of your input and that of the speech and language service in general, and any relevant information that you have about the client. This exchange of information and liaison may take place through:

- informal discussion among staff
- attendance on ward rounds
- notes kept in the patient's medical file
- information kept in the nurses' Cardex/care plan system
- liaison with the primary nurse or key worker involved with the client
- letters and reports sent to referring agents, etc.
- case conferences and ward meetings.

The speech and language clinicians should clarify where their own contact should be recorded on the ward, so that other members of the team are aware of their involvement.

The ward setting

The hospital ward is invariably a busy place with many different profes-sionals, all needing to carry out important tasks in relation to the patient. It is important that, as the speech and language clinician, you make yourself known to the person with day-to-day responsibility for the ward. This is usually the charge nurse or sister. You should then negotiate a suitable time and space to work with the patient. Many wards now have unrestricted visiting so you must be sensitive to the needs of family and friends.

Private space is often at a premium, so some consultations may need to take place at the bedside, with maybe only a curtain between the patient and the rest of the ward. This can be quite a distracting environment and there may be little privacy for confidential case history taking and personal discussion.

Some patients, particularly if they are required to spend more than a few days in hospital, may become somewhat 'institutionalized' by the process. Signs of this may include:

- passivity and over-compliance
- the inability to make decisions
- depression and lack of motivation.

This is likely to have consequences on their response to any intervention and may give a false impression of their attitudes to communication and recovery.

The outpatient department

Here the clinician may have more control over the timing of appointments for both clients who are inpatients and may be brought from the ward, and clients who are outpatients and may require ambulance or hospital transport. However, these clients may still be involved with a number of hospital personnel and there may be a need for careful scheduling so that they do not have to make unnecessary trips to the hospital.

There are several points to consider:

- Can a joint appointment with other therapy staff be made, e.g. coordinated with physiotherapy or occupational therapy?
- Can the client cope with this level of input or is this too fatiguing?
- Is the order of appointments important? For example, relaxation carried out by the physiotherapist may have positive effects on the subsequent speech and language programme.
- Is this the most effective setting for therapy or would the client be more responsive if he or she was seen at home?

Within the outpatient department, the speech and language clinician is likely to have access to a greater variety of materials and a quieter environment for assessment and confidential discussion than on the ward. However, more effort may be needed to liaise with other staff and to keep ward notes up to date.

Domiciliary visits

How much opportunity the speech and language clinician will have to undertake domiciliary visits will depend on:

- the policy of the department
- the geographical area
- the facilities available within the hospital
- the need for specialist equipment available only within the department
- the experience and level of supervision required by the therapist
- safety considerations.

The home environment may hold advantages for the client and provides the opportunity for you, the therapist, to:

- see clients when they are relaxed and at the best time of day
- observe the clients' communication skills in a functional setting
- have close contact with relatives and carers
- plan intervention that is relevant to the clients' everyday needs and environment.

However, you need to be aware of the additional time and organization that may be needed to travel round the locality and the necessity of having the materials that you need for assessment and intervention with the clients. You also need to be aware of the potential risk that may be involved with seeing clients away from a centre where there are other staff on hand. Before undertaking a domiciliary visit you should:

- consider the level of potential risk involved with a particular client or setting and undertake a risk assessment
- check the department policy in relation to domiciliary visits or 'lone worker' and discuss this with the manager, and have appropriate lone worker training
- carry and wear an identification badge
- consider whether the planned procedure may pose a potential risk to the client, e.g. an assessment for dysphagia
- be aware of safety procedures relevant to home visits, e.g. dealing with challenging behaviour or medical emergencies
- make sure that someone at the base knows where they are visiting and, if necessary, arrange to contact the base on completion of the visit
- where necessary, arrange to visit with a colleague or another professional.

Child development centre

These centres provide a central focus for the assessment, or assessment and treatment, of children with complex needs. These teams are usually coordinated by a consultant paediatrician, will also have input from a range of therapists and a clinical psychologist, and may include representatives from social services and education. Most children seen at these centres are likely to be below the age of 5 years, although some centres also cater for school-aged children.

The multidisciplinary assessment

Instead of having to visit several different professionals for individual appointments, the child and his or her family may be offered an extended appointment when all the relevant professionals may be available. Once the assessment has been completed, there will be a multiprofessional conference, including the parents, at which a coordinated plan of care and therapy will be agreed. This therapy may take place within the child development centre (CDC), again limiting the number of appointments that the family has to keep. In some centres the recommendations of the team will be passed on to local clinicians so that intervention takes place in the child's locality, but with the supervision and support of the specialist team. Many centres may also run multidisciplinary groups where, for example, speech and language therapy, physiotherapy and other disciplines provide input to a group of children attending the same session.

This setting can also provide the child's parents with the opportunity to meet and talk with other families who may be experiencing similar problems, and may be a useful source of general advice and information for the community clinician. The Special Educational Needs Statementing process may begin at this time, so that suitable school placement can be planned.

Rehabilitation centres

These centres are designed to provide intensive therapeutic rehabilitation, and clients may either be residential or attend on a daily basis. The main aims of the service are to help clients to reach their full potential and to maximize long-term functioning. Referral to the centre is usually via medical personnel and the centre is likely to be managed by a consultant. As well as in-depth assessment of communication and swallowing disorders, the speech and language clinician may be involved with other disciplines in the assessment of related skills, e.g.:

- Speech and language therapy (SLT) and physiotherapy: posture, breathing and voice production
- SLT and occupational therapy: writing and accessing of augmentative and alternative communication (AAC) devices
- SLT and psychologist: cognition, reasoning, memory skills.

Following the multidisciplinary assessment, a joint report and care plan will be drawn up by the team in consultation with the client and his or her carers. This plan may then be carried out within the rehabilitation centre where intensive therapy input can be arranged, or less intensive therapy may be arranged on an outpatient or domiciliary basis.

Community clinics/health centres

The health centre is the base for members of the PCT. This is usually the client's first and main access to health services.

This team is usually coordinated by the GP, who will be the gatekeeper to a range of other services, including referral to specialist medical personnel. The PCT has responsibility for purchasing health care from health-care providers. Their budget is allocated from central government on a per capita basis. It is essential that GPs be kept informed of the speech and language clinician's involvement with their clients; this can be done through copies of letters to acknowledge referral, reports written after assessment, and interim and discharge reports.

Although, in theory, any client may access speech and language services through their local health centre, in practice most health centre/clinic referrals will be pre-school children. In some areas children may continue to be seen at their local clinic after they have started school, whereas in other areas they are likely to have their management transferred to a clinician who visits and works in their school. Some community clinicians may be happy to assess and work with a wider client group, e.g. adults with learning disabilities and adults discharged from hospital, but less experienced staff may wish to pass these referrals on to the relevant specialists.

Personnel working in hospitals, clinics and health centres

Primary care

The general practitioner

The GP will be the leader of the primary care team and will be responsible for all decisions made about the patients on his or her list. He or she is an important source of information and referral. *Health for All Children* (Hall and Elliman 2003) has outlined arrangements for routine, evidence-based screening of babies and young children by GPs, which may lead to referral for speech and language assessment.

The health visitor

This is a fully qualified nurse who has undergone additional training. She or he may work particularly with young families. The role of the health visitor is developing into a more proactive approach to the promotion of health. Their involvement is likely to focus on screening as a result of parental concern and follow-up of children who fail to thrive. As this practice becomes more established, it may well impact on how and when children are referred to a speech and language service. However, the health visitor's regular contact with families means that she or he is frequently the primary referring agency for pre-school children to the speech and language service, and will usually be able to provide detailed background information on the child and family. The emphasis of their work is moving towards a health promotion role, working as part of the multidisciplinary team supporting the child and family.

The practice nurse

As well as carrying out routine nursing activities within the centre, the practice nurse may run special clinics for particular groups of patients with conditions such as diabetes and asthma. The practice nurse can be an extremely useful source of information about particular patients, and needs to be kept informed of the clinician's involvement.

The district nurse

The district nurse will provide nursing care and support to people in their homes, and may be a useful source of information. She or he may be particularly involved with a patient immediately after discharge from hospital and will be aware of social as well as medical aspects of the patient's condition.

The community nurse

The community nurse will usually have specific training in relation to learning disability or mental health issues. She or he will be a primary point of contact and support for the clients and their families, and will also provide information on medical needs, financial benefits and local resources and, where appropriate, will arrange for referral to other relevant professionals. There may also be designated nurses who are specialists in dealing with particular client groups, such as those presenting with challenging behaviour.

The practice manager

Practice managers are responsible for the day-to-day running of the health centre, and will organize such things as room availability, resources, security, admin support, etc. If the clinician is based within the clinic, it is important to negotiate access and keep the manager informed of her or his activities.

Secondary care

The clinical director

This may be a doctor, nurse or member of the paramedical professions who heads up the clinical directorate and who will have both clinical and managerial responsibilities. The clinical director may have responsibility for a number of different professionals within the directorate and will represent their views to the chief executive.

Consultant

This is the most senior doctor working within the hospital, who will ultimately be responsible for the patient's medical care. He or she will be a specialist in his or her particular area of medicine, e.g. orthopaedics, oncology or geriatric medicine. He or she may be the source of referral of in- or outpatients and will need to be kept fully informed of the clinician's involvement. The consultant will be supported by junior doctors, such as senior registrars and house officers, who are training to become consultants or GPs.

Medical officer

There will be a designated officer for special educational needs who will coordinate the strategic and operational activity relating to these. This will include coordinating the school health service and health advice for the statutory assessment. Requests for Statement advice will be sent to a medical officer whose role will be to ensure that all other relevant health professionals are consulted.

Nursing staff

Charge nurse/sister
This is the person responsible for the day-to-day care of the patients on her or his ward. She or he is responsible for the allocation of nursing duties and the overall organization of ward staff.

Primary nurse
In many hospitals the patient will be assigned a primary nurse who takes responsibility for a named group of patients. She or he will be responsible for coordinating the patient's care and liaising with relatives and other professionals as necessary.

Other health-care staff who may work in a range of settings are the following.

Physiotherapists

Physiotherapists use special skills and techniques to help people who are physically disabled by injury or illness to achieve as normal and active a life as possible. They may work in hospitals, health centres, clinics, schools or people's homes, and they provide a service to all ages.

Occupational therapists

The aim of occupational therapists is to help people to achieve and maintain the maximum degree of independence possible in all aspects of their daily lives. This may involve teaching different ways of doing everyday tasks, supplying special equipment, recommending adaptation to housing, etc. They work with all age ranges and may be employed within the health service or by the Social Services department.

Dietitians

Dietitians may work within the hospital or be based in the community. They aim to promote health and prevent disease by giving dietary and nutritional advice to patients and staff. They are likely to be involved in the management of children and adults with swallowing difficulties, and can advise on suitable textures and food supplements.

Clinical psychologists

Clinical psychologists are trained in the assessment and treatment of psychological problems. They provide a service for people of all ages with a wide range of health problems, in particular those with learning disabilities, elderly people, and children and adults with mental health problems. Their aim is to help people to develop more effective ways of coping with problems and illness, and in the management of problem behaviour.

Administrative staff

Such individuals will be a vital source of information and may be responsible for some of the clinician's administration tasks, such as typing reports, sending out appointments, etc. In some situations all administration will go through a central speech and language office. No matter where the clinician is based, it is important that a member of staff be aware of her activities at all times. This is for her own personal safety, e.g. if she undertakes a home visit she should let someone know where she is and at what time she should be expected back. The receptionist will also be the first line of contact for her clients and should therefore have the information needed to keep clients informed.

The education context

In some areas speech and language clinicians may be employed directly by the education department or school. However, in the UK, speech and language services in schools may be provided by the local NHS Trust, although increasingly Trusts and local education authorities (LEAs) are entering into joint funding arrangements. Here the NHS Trust may retain overall responsibility for a service that is partly financed by the education department. However, it is recognized that there is often a significant short-fall between the amount of therapy provided and what the LEA would like (Council of Local Education Authorities 1994). More recently, the Department of Education and Skills (DfES) has made money available through Standards Funds (Department of Education and Science 2000) to develop national priorities. In many areas this funding has been used to increase speech and language therapy provision in schools. This has resulted in services and clinicians developing innovative working practices and a greater cooperation with school staff.

There has been considerable change to the organization of the education system in the UK, as a result of a range of legislation since the late 1980s:

1. 1988: The Education Reform Act – this far-reaching legislation involved:
   - the implementation of the National Curriculum, and national assessment arrangements – Standard Assessment Tasks (SATs)
   - the introduction of local management of schools (LMS), which gives schools greater budgetary and decision-making control
   - an increase in the powers and responsibilities of school governors
   - the introduction of open enrolment, allowing parents greater choice over school placement.
2. 1992: the Office for Standards in Education (OFSTED) was set up to inspect, report and improve the standards of achievement and quality in schools by a 4-year cycle of school inspection. Also, school league tables were introduced and published allowing parents to compare school attainment and examination results.

3. 1993: the Funding Agency for Schools in England, the Schools Funding Council for Wales and the Education Committee of the Scottish Parliament were established, to take over responsibility for planning school places within their areas.

4. 1996: legislation was introduced to raise the standards in schools by encouraging schools to take greater responsibility for achieving high standards, by setting targets and accounting for performance. This included an extension of LMS so that schools control 95 per cent of the budget, although the financing of children with Statements of Educational Need/Record of Need still remains with the LEA.

5. 1997: a consultative paper was published that aimed to increase inclusion of children with special educational needs. It also sought to provide speech and language therapy more effectively for the children who needed it and encouraged the more effective and widespread use of information and communication technology to support their education.

6. 2001: the Special Educational Needs and Disability Act ensured that discrimination against disabled students would be unlawful and supported greater inclusion within mainstream schools, and the Special Educational Needs: Code of Practice Conduct 2001 outlined the assessment and planning process.

7. 2004: removing barriers to achievement widened opportunities in mainstream school, promoted greater 'inclusion' of pupils with special needs and transformed special schools.

In relation to children with special needs, the 1981 Education Act provided the foundation for services for children with special needs in the UK. A child is viewed as having special educational needs if:

> he has a learning difficulty which calls for special educational provision to be made for him . . . and a child has a 'learning difficulty' if . . . he has a significantly greater difficulty in learning than the majority of children of his age.
>
> Department of Education and Science (1981, p. 6)

The Warnock Report (Department of Education and Science 1978), the precursor to the 1981 Act, suggested that between 18 and 20 per cent of children would have some sort of special educational need at some stage of their school career. At this time special schools were catering for about 2 per cent of the school population.

Other aspects of the Act promoted an integrated education service for these children, and introduced the concept of the 'Statement of Educational Need' in England and Wales. A similar process exists in Scotland; here children have a 'Record of Need'. These are legal documents drawn up by the LEA in consultation with parents and the professionals involved with the child. They outline the child's special educational needs and the resources necessary to meet these needs. As a result of this legislation and the commitment to a policy of integration, some special schools closed and most of the others underwent a significant change in their character and organization. However, the Warnock Committee envisaged that there would always be a small core of children who would require segregated school provision. From the 1980s, there was a steady rise in the number of children being given the protection of a Statement, although the number of these in special school had dropped to 1.1 per cent by 2004. However, there is a very varied national picture, with some local authorities providing Statements for less than 1.5 per cent of their pupils, and other LEAs statementing well over 5 per cent of the school population (Table 6.1).

Table 6.1 Numbers of children in England with a Statement of Educational Need

Year	Number
1994	184 245
1996	216 546
1998	231 139
2000	241 434
2001	247 200

Although the principles introduced by the 1981 Act have been maintained, the process has been revised by the introduction of the Code of Practice on the Identification and Assessment of Special Educational Needs (DfES 2001). This clearly outlines the assessment and statementing procedure, and identifies the school's and the LEA's responsibilities in relation to this process. All children should have a recorded 'individual education plan' (IEP), which defines the targets for learning (Table 6.2). It also aims to limit the issuing of a Statement to those children who require resources beyond those usually available in the mainstream school. The purpose is to focus resources on the 2 per cent of children who have severe and/or complex needs. The Code of Practice also outlines appeals and tribunal procedures for parents who are unhappy with the decisions made by the LEA. The Code was further revised in 2001 to strengthen the child's right to be educated in mainstream school, increase pupil participation and provide clearer guidelines for early years' education. Since 2000 educational pre-school settings have undertaken a Foundation Stage assessment to provide a profile that can help with the early identification of children who may require additional support. *Removing Barriers to Achievement* (DfES 2004) has further strengthened the right of the child to be educated in a mainstream setting, and outlines guidance to ensure 'inclusion'.

The Warnock Report (Department of Education and Science 1978) was keen to abolish categories of disability and replace them with an overarching

Table 6.2 Progression of support for children with additional learning needs

Differentiation of the curriculum: the adjustment of the National Curriculum to meet the needs of children functioning at different levels. This is part of good classroom management. 'P Scales' are available for children where the early levels of the National Curriculum are not appropriate. These are performance descriptors for measuring progression. They include separate strands for speaking and listening

School action: class teacher provides interventions that are additional or different from schools' usual differentiated curriculum; strategies employed should be recorded in an individual educational plan (IEP)

School action plus: external support services will become involved with the child, to give advice on new IEPs

Statutory assessment: leading to a Statement or note in lieu of statement

Statement: summarizes special educational needs, and proposed provision and placement

Annual review: all Statements must be reviewed at least annually, and amendments made to the statement as required

definition of learning disability. Guidance now accepts that there are no hard-and-fast categories of special education need, and that each child will have his or her unique profile of strengths and special needs. However, these are likely to fall into the following areas:

- **Communication and interaction**: this will include children with speech and language delay or disorder, specific learning difficulties such as dyslexia and dyspraxia, hearing impairment or autistic spectrum disorders.
- **Cognition and learning**: this may include children with moderate, severe or profound learning difficulties.
- **Behaviour, emotional and social development**: children with challenging behaviour, hyperactivity and immature social skills.
- **Sensory and/or physical needs**.
- **Medical conditions**.

Children with speech and language difficulties in mainstream education

There are likely to be a number of children in mainstream schools who will require the attention of a speech and language clinician. They can be divided into two groups.

Statemented children

These will usually be the children with the more severe and complex needs, who have undergone the full assessment process. Their Statement will usually be related to problems with communication and interaction. Many of these children will have severe communication difficulties and may require the input of a speech and language clinician. Case law has established that speech and language therapy can be considered as either educational or non-educational provision. However, as communication is viewed as fundamental to the education process it should be recorded under educational provision unless there are exceptional reasons for not doing so (Special Educational Needs: Code of Practice – DfES 2001). It is important that the speech and language clinician working in schools is fully conversant with current education legislation, and that she consider the educational implications of the child's communication difficulties.

Non-Statemented children

Many children with communication difficulties will not fall into this 2 per cent, and the educational needs of these children will have to be met by the resources available within the school. Some speech and language services have a policy of providing help and support to all schoolchildren within the school setting. Others will provide support only to those children in possession of a Statement, with other children being catered for as clients at their local community clinic or health centre.

Children with speech and language difficulties in special schools

Although there has been a drive to promote 'inclusive education', it is recognized that some children may benefit from being in a specialist environment, and parents may choose to send their child to a special school. These schools usually cater for children with the most severe and complex needs. The schools may have regular and/or intensive support from a speech and language clinician.

Speech and language intervention within the school

When you are working in a school on a regular basis, it is important that you, as well as everyone else, are clear about how such working will be arranged. It is useful to meet the headteacher and special needs coordinator (SENCO) to negotiate arrangements before the block of visits begins. For inexperienced staff it is useful to have a more senior speech and language clinician or manager present at this initial meeting. The areas that need to be discussed include the following:

- With whom will you be working:
  - all children with speech and language problems?
  - only those with Statements?
- How will new referrals be handled?
- What do school staff expect of you? Is this realistic?
- What do you expect of school staff? Again, is this realistic?
- Where will you work?

- When will you be in school?
- Who will be your main point of contact and liaison?
  - the SENCO
  - an assistant
  - the headteacher.
- How will your work be integrated into the classroom?
- When will you be able to meet school staff to discuss individual children?
- Who will be responsible for carryover work and implementing programmes?

It is useful to document these decisions and provide all interested partners with a copy, so that there can be no misunderstandings about these key issues. This does not mean that the arrangements cannot be changed, but such change should be done through a process of consultation on both sides, rather than by decisions being made unilaterally.

Roulstone (1986) suggests that the speech and language clinician fulfils at least three distinct roles within a school:

1. Coordinator of all aspects of communication: this may involve coordinating language groups, work with assistants and other personnel.
2. Skills transmitter: this may be done on a one-to-one basis in the classroom, or through more formalized training sessions, such as teaching sign language to all staff in school.
3. Participant: it is important that the clinician is seen as an integral part of the work environment. It may be important to participate in a wide range of curricular and extracurricular activities. This will enable her or him to model and encourage appropriate communication strategies and establish credibility with the team.

The main roles of the speech and language clinician within the school are likely to include:

- assessment
- direct intervention
- provision of programmes
- team teaching, group work and modelling strategies within the classroom
- staff and parental training
- contribution to school policies.

Assessment

The communication and eating and drinking difficulties of many children may have been identified in the pre-school years. However, there is likely to be a number of children whose speech and language problems have not become apparent until they have been exposed to the challenges of the classroom situation. This may be because they have been able to establish good interaction with familiar adults, or their difficulties in intelligibility may arise only when they are in a situation where they have to communicate with less familiar people. For some children, language difficulties may be revealed when they begin to struggle with some of the speaking and listening targets of the National Curriculum, or when they have difficulty with the development of early reading and writing skills. Another group often not identified until they reach school age is children with pragmatic difficulties who may exhibit great difficulty establishing peer relationships.

For these reasons, you, as the speech and language clinician working in schools, can expect to receive a number of new referrals of children who will need assessment. It is important that parents have given clear consent to the referral before any involvement by you with the child. It is good practice to seek the parents' views and feelings about their child's difficulty by inviting them, wherever possible, to be a part of the assessment process.

There will also be a need for ongoing assessment and reassessment of children as they progress though the school system. The Code of Practice requires an IEP to be in place for any child experiencing difficulty in the classroom. This should include aims and objectives relating to speech, language and communication development and will need to be reviewed and revised on a regularly basis (see example in Figure 6.3).

Any child who is the subject of a school-based IEP or Statement of Educational Need will have their progress reviewed and monitored on a regular basis, and at least annually. The speech and language clinician will be required to provide reports on the child's progress in communication and will be invited to participate in the annual review meeting.

Direct intervention

There is likely to be a small number of children with whom you may wish to work directly on a regular basis. Even when most of the intervention is being carried out by others, it will still be important to monitor progress directly in some way. There will thus always remain a need to work directly with the client on some occasions:

- for further assessment
- for review and report writing
- at the request of other team members
- when the clinician is unsure about how to proceed with the client
- to demonstrate procedures and techniques to others
- when using specific equipment and techniques
- to maintain a relationship with the client
- to establish credibility within the team.

NAME: John B.	YEAR: 2

Language and communication: (including English)
1. Develop John's reading skills to a point where his reading age is within 2 years of his chronological age

2. Increase his understanding of instructions incorporating 4 or more information-carrying words

Academic development (including maths, science and foundation subjects)
Count and give amounts of money up to £5

Visuo-motor development
Hits a tennis ball thrown from 3 metres, with a flat bat 6/10 times

Social and emotional development
1. Relay verbal messages to others within school
2. Play a board game with another child for at least 5 minutes without adult intervention

Notes
A programme will be provided by the speech and language therapist, and implemented three times a week by the SNA

Medical factors
John's epilepsy is being monitored. All staff should be advised of what to do in case of a fit

Teacher's name: **Date:**

Signature:

Figure 6.3 An individual education plan.

On some occasions you may wish to withdraw children into a quiet one-to-one situation. Increasingly, however, visiting professionals are recognizing the value of working in the child's natural environment, rather than working in an isolated one-to-one setting (the traditional broom cupboard). The benefits of working within the classroom include:

- assessing and identifying the child's strengths and weaknesses in a more natural educational setting
- aims and objectives being more likely to be relevant to the child's everyday needs
- therapy being seen as part of the total educational process and made relevant to the classroom activities and environment
- involving other personnel more easily in the programme and the clinician modelling appropriate strategies

- similarly the clinician being exposed to the strategies of other personnel (e.g. in relation to behaviour management)
- the clinician also being likely to be made aware of the pressures experienced within a busy classroom, so she or he can tailor her or his demands accordingly
- language skills more likely to be generalized if they are integrated into the environment where natural cues occur.

McCartney (1999) identified a number of barriers to collaboration between teachers and speech and language clinicians, including:

- Functional barriers, in particular definition of for whom a service is provided and models of interprofessional interaction
- Structural barriers relating to the formalized interactions between services and management structures
- Process barriers – differences between educational and health-care processes.

Teachers are always keen to welcome other professionals into the classroom. A survey by Gipps et al. (1987) investigated teachers' attitudes to the range of support being provided for children with special needs in mainstream classrooms. They found that withdrawal by specially trained staff was viewed more favourably than assistance in the classroom or in-service training. It was felt that this was partly a reflection of previously established working practices, but also indicated a feeling of a lack of experience and expertise in dealing with these children. There was also a reluctance to accept responsibility for their needs. There has been a considerable investment in in-service training and changes in attitudes during the past few years, e.g. Invalid Children's Association Nationwide (I-CAN 2004) has produced a framework for joint post-registration training *Learning Together: Working Together*, for teachers and speech and language clinicians working in early years' settings.

Visiting professionals must be sensitive to the teacher's situation. They should be aware of their lack of in-depth training and experience in communication, the demands of a large and diverse class, and the range of other responsibilities of the class teacher. Working practice should be clearly discussed and sensitively negotiated between all personnel involved. Finally, it should not be forgotten that there may be advantages to withdrawing the child from the classroom on some occasions:

- It provides an opportunity for the child to spend time with an adult in what may be a more relaxed and less stressful environment.
- Some children may be very sensitive to failing in front of their peers, so may be reluctant to experiment with new skills within the classroom.
- A child with attention difficulties may need the opportunity to work in a quiet environment on some occasions.

- Assessment to compare 'optimum' ability with 'functional' ability may be useful.
- Some procedures (e.g. oral examinations) may need to be done in a private setting to preserve dignity.
- The therapist may be unsure of a procedure and may need to experiment in a less open environment.
- A procedure may require the use of specialist equipment unsuitable to the classroom environment.
- Certain therapy procedures may be highly distracting and not appropriate to the classroom setting.
- Likewise, some class activities may not be conducive to focusing on the needs of one particular child.

Provision of programmes to be carried out by school personnel

Increasingly, speech and language clinicians are working within a consultative model in schools, where they may have much less 'hands on' experience than was traditionally the case. This requires the development of a different range of skills, and success is dependent on good interpersonal relationships and the ability to negotiate with all involved. If the child has the protection of a Statement this may include the allocation of extra teaching or non-teaching assistance. This may even be specified as time for speech and language activities. Without a Statement to define such support, time to carry out communication programmes may be at the expense of other activities and will be very much at the discretion of school staff. However the time is arranged, it is important that it can be used as effectively and efficiently as possible. This means that any programme must be easy to implement and the materials must be readily available (Figures 6.4 and 6.5).

Staff training

Teachers may be involved in a range of both school-based and external in-service training. It is now quite common practice for speech and language clinicians to run training courses for special needs assistants, SENCOs and other interested staff. This is seen as a way to provide information and develop skills, as well as changing attitudes and building good working relationships, e.g. Elklan-SLT in the Classroom training (Elks and McLachlan 2004).

School staff are expected to have a commitment to attending a set number of staff development sessions during the year. Many schools will run in-service training (inset) days, where the speech and language clinician may contribute as either presenter or participant. Other informal training may take place through ongoing involvement with staff in the classroom setting. These situations can also give the speech and language clinician greater understanding of current educational issues and school policies, as well as building on her or his relationship with the school staff.

A programme should include:
Summary of present skills This can be used to highlight current or newly acquired skills as a foundation for the present aims
Clear aims These should be written in easily understandable language that relates to activities already going on in the classroom. For example, if the class is covering a particular science topic, make sure that the programme is focusing on the same vocabulary and concepts
Context It may be helpful to specify the setting in which activities should take place, i.e. group, quiet corner, etc.
Materials needed If you are not able to supply these, make sure the assistant has a full list of everything that will be needed before the activity is begun. It may be useful to have them collected together in a clearly labelled box or corner
Procedures/suggested activities You will need to provide a range of activities for each aim, so that there is variety for both the child and the assistant
Reinforcement/feedback How should this be incorporated into the activity? It needs to be simple and quick so that it is done on a routine basis
Record keeping This needs to be a quick and easily managed process, which documents the input and progress of the child
General considerations This would include suggestions for how to encourage carry over new skills into other contexts
Review What should be done in case of difficulties? How can you be contacted? It should also include an indication of when the programme will be reviewed

Figure 6.4 Guidelines for writing a programme.

NAME: Lisa M.   D.O.B.: 8/8/92   C.A: 6:1
SCHOOL: Whitegates Special School   DATE: 12/9/97
<u>Summary of present communication</u> Lisa is beginning to use language appropriately but needs to extend her organization of language and language concepts
<u>Aims of programme</u> 1. To develop her understanding of instructions containing four information-carrying words, e.g. Give the <u>little cow</u> a <u>big cup</u>. 2. To develop her ability to give instructions containing three elements, e.g. put the <u>car</u> <u>under</u> the <u>table</u>.

Figure 6.5 Example of a programme.   (contd)

Context
Lisa is easily distracted, so it will help her to work in a quiet, distraction-free environment

Materials needed
1. A set of large and small everyday objects and a large and small box and bag
2. Large and small dolls and teddies
3. Symbol pictures
4. Farmyard picture, and two sets of identical farm animals

Suggested activities
1. Give L. instructions about where to put the objects away, e.g. 'Put the big spoon in the big box'. Take it in turns so L. then asks you to put something away, using the name of the object and its location. Try to discourage her from just pointing. When she is giving you instructions you may need to simplify it so she only labels the object rather that thinking about the size, e.g. 'Put the spoon in the big bag'

2. Direct L. to carry out a range of actions, e.g. 'Wash the big teddy's feet', 'Put little teddy under the table'. Again try role-reversal so she then gives you directions as to what she wants

3. Take it in turns to colour in, e.g. 'Make the little pig red'

4. Try a barrier-type game involving another child, where you use a screen or box so you can't see what each other has done. Set the animals around the farm for L. She has to tell the other child what to do to make hers the same, e.g. 'The cow is next to the house, the duck is on the pond'. Then change them over so that the other child gives the directions to L. The adult will need to help to make sure they do this orally, rather than be pointing

If L. enjoys this type of activity I'm sure you will come up with lots of other ideas

Reinforcement/feedback
L. should find most of these activities rewarding in their own right, but remember to give her verbal encouragement and model the correct response if she is having difficulty

Record-keeping
Please can you complete the attached form to give me feedback on the activities

General considerations
Once L. is feeling confident with these types of tasks it may be helpful to incorporate them into 'circle time' with the whole class group

Review
This programme will be reviewed again in January 1999, but please contact me before then if you require any further ideas or support

Signed

Figure 6.5 (contd)

Input into school policies and curriculum development

Finally, speech and language clinicians can be seen as a resource in relation to speech and language development. They may be able to contribute to more general aspects of the language curriculum, and in particular the speaking and listening components of the National Curriculum. Speech and language clinicians should make themselves aware of the policies in operation in the schools in which they are working. This may include policies on:

- language and literacy
- child protection
- dealing with challenging behaviour
- mealtime management.

The majority of speech and language therapy input is likely to be during the primary school years, but there will be a small core of children who may continue to need support when they move to secondary education. The organization of this will need to be sensitively handled so that the child is not stigmatized by the experience, or withdrawn from important subject areas.

Further education

In recent years, there has been a growth in the number of further education courses catering for individuals with learning disabilities or autistic spectrum disorders. This may be a specific full-time course designed to help with the transition from school to adult life, or clients may access a range of individual adult education classes. These may include academic skills, such as literacy, language and numeracy, or may provide access to leisure activities. Speech and language clinicians may be involved in supporting individuals in their transition from school to college or may contribute to communication aspects of a particular course.

Personnel

The headteacher

It should be remembered that the head is in overall charge of the school and should be kept informed of the clinician's contact with the children in the school. They are 'in loco parentis' and therefore ultimately responsible for the child while he or she is on the school premises.

The special educational needs coordinator

Each school has an appointed SENCO who has responsibility for implementing the school's special educational needs policy and monitoring children on the Special Needs Register. He or she will also be involved in supporting staff with the assessment process, developing IEPs and providing teaching support. His or her role will also be to liaise with external professionals. In many cases the SENCO may be the main point of contact for the speech and language clinician.

The class teacher

Although initial contact may be made through the SENCO, it is important to remember that the class teacher is responsible for the day-to-day management of the child and should be kept involved with the speech and language programme. The availability of the child, work in the classroom, etc., should be negotiated directly with the class teacher.

The teaching assistant

Some individual children may have a full- or part-time assistant appointed as part of their Statement of Educational Need. These assistants will have a clearly defined role within the classroom in relation to this child, and this may include speech and language therapy support. Other assistants may be appointed to support a group or class of children, but may be able to follow up on speech and language programmes with specific children. The role of 'higher-level teaching assistants' is currently being developed. These experienced staff may have skills in specific areas such as dyslexia or AAC support, and will take on greater responsibility in the classroom.

The child protection coordinator

Schools should also have an appointed member of staff with responsibility for child protection issues. This person should be the clinician's first point of contact if she has any concerns about a child. The coordinator is responsible for contact with outside agencies while the child is at school.

The school nurse

Some special schools, especially those catering for children with physical disabilities, may have the regular services of a school nurse who will be responsible for medication and health care, e.g. supervising gastrostomy feeds. All mainstream schools will have a designated school nurse who may cover several schools in the area. The nurse can be a useful source of information and can arrange medical checks on request.

The advisory teacher

LEAs may employ a number of advisory teachers to provide support to schools in the area. This support is usually provided to the teaching staff in terms of resources and advice, but may also involve assessment and direct interaction with the child. Advisory teachers may include specialist teachers for visually impaired children, hearing impaired children, information technology, etc.

The educational psychologist

The educational psychologist will have a key role to play in the decision-making process and in many cases will be responsible for the coordination of the formal statement process. He or she will also give advice to teachers on educational and behavioural management.

The social welfare context

Speech and language clinicians may work in a range of settings that are organized and funded by the local authority Social Services department. They may also liaise with casework social workers in relation to specific clients in their care.

Residential and day services for children, individuals with disabilities and older people

Domiciliary and residential care

Care (Table 6.3) is provided for anyone over the age of 18 who needs it because of age, disability or illness. Where possible, support will be provided to enable individuals to remain in their own home. Support may include regular help with personal care, meals at home and help with adaptations to the house. The provision of this service is means tested, and will be closely linked to informal care provided by friends and relatives. The care assistant is a vital link between the client and other services, and can provide support as well as monitoring changes in the client's health and well-being.

Short-term residential care may be arranged to give carers a break, or to help get people back on their feet after a period in hospital. If an individual is assessed and needs a care package, he or she may qualify for direct payments. This scheme makes regular monthly payments to enable individuals to employ their own personal assistants, and provides greater freedom and control. On occasions, it may be necessary to provide long-term 24-hour care. This is provided in care homes (formerly known as residential homes) and care homes with nursing (formerly nursing homes). Since the introduction of the NHS and Community Care Act 1990 much of this care is provided by the private sector and is the result of a full assessment of need. Social Services will provide an assessment and will advise about the cost of care, and what the individual will be liable to pay. Some facilities are still run by Social Services and they remain responsible for the overall inspection and approval of residential services.

Table 6.3 Residential care

	Acute emergency care	Rehabilitation/continuing care
Home-based	Intensive home support Emergency duty teams Sector teams	Domiciliary services Key workers Care management
Day care	Day hospitals	Drop-in centres Support groups Employment schemes Day care
Residential support	Crisis accommodation Acute units Local secure units	Ordinary housing Unstaffed group homes Adult placement schemes Residential care homes Mental nursing homes 24-hour NHS accommodation Medium secure units High security units

DoH (1993: 71).

Some NHS trust policies do not provide for therapy input into privately run homes. Other managers argue that the residential establishment is the client's home and so they should be provided with the same domiciliary support as those people still residing in their own homes. It is important to check the department policy before arranging to visit. As well as working with individual clients in this setting, the speech and language clinician may organize group therapy, such as setting up 'reminiscence groups'. They may also provide advice and training around communication and/or eating and drinking difficulties.

Day centres

Services are also provided in day centres, which may be totally funded by Social Services or a joint initiative with health trusts. Here the speech and language clinician may work with both individuals and groups and provide regular training for staff. Day centres commonly cater for the older person, adults with learning disabilities or mental health problems, and people with physical disabilities. There is increasing diversity in the range of options available. Person-centred planning is a process where the individual is enabled to define what services he or she requires.

Care management

Where the needs of a client are complex or involve significant resources, the Social Services department will need to arrange for an assessment of need.

The care manager will arrange for this assessment and help to draw up a care plan. The role of the care manager is then to procure the resources and services outlined in the plan and to monitor and review its implementation; they are not responsible for the provision of these services. Care may be purchased from a range of statutory, voluntary and private agencies. The core tasks of care management are:

- publication of information about available resources
- determination of the level of assessment needed
- assessment of need
- care planning
- implementation of the care plan
- monitoring
- reviewing.

Adults with learning disabilities

The concept of 'normalization' or 'social role valorization' emerged from the USA in the 1970s and has significantly altered attitudes and provision for adults with learning disabilities. Foxen and McBrien (1981) describe five key values for a service promoting 'ordinary life' values:

1. Community presence: provision of both residential and day services within the community.
2. Competence: the development of skills in order to participate in the local community.
3. Choice: promotion of a range of options and opportunities.
4. Respect: service should help people to enjoy the same status as other valued members of society.
5. Relationships: service should help and encourage individuals to mix with other non-disabled people.

The Valuing People White Paper (DoH 2001a) defined services for this group for the twenty-first century. This highlights the need for development in the following areas:

- Services to children and young people
- Increased choice and control and the implementation of person-centred planning
- Support for carers
- Improved health
- Housing, employment and leisure options
- The development of quality services – through workforce planning and education.

Increasingly, speech and language clinicians are involved in the development of services for this client group. The Royal College of Speech and

Language Therapists' (RCSLT's) Position Paper (RCSLT 2003b) identifies three distinct roles for the specialist:

1. Specialist clinical skills: including specialist assessment and intervention.
2. Facilitation of others: through education and training.
3. Service development: involvement with policy development and cultural change.

Individual programme planning

A coordinator will usually be appointed to support the client and collect together information that will be presented at the individual programme planning (IPP) meeting. This information will focus on the client's strengths and needs. Areas considered may include:

• basic physical skills
• communication skills
• self-care and domestic skills
• recreation and leisure skills and opportunities
• social skills and personal relationships
• medical and financial needs.

At the meeting this information will be considered, and a plan of goals agreed with the client will be drawn up. Clear decisions will be made and documented about who will take responsibility for each part of this programme. This plan will be reviewed as part of subsequent annual IPP meetings.

Person-centred planning

This is a process where the service user is helped to define and voice his or her aspirations. Services should then explore how they can facilitate the realization of these plans. This means that provision should be person-centred and not based purely on a needs assessment or designed around what services are currently available.

Supported living/group homes

This move to the community has involved considerable changes in the philosophy and working practices of staff involved. The speech and language clinician must be able to respond in a flexible manner to the training needs of staff as well as the therapy needs of the clients. However, it should be remembered that most adults with learning disabilities continue to live with their families, who may also require a range of different kinds of help and support.

Day care provision

Social education centres/adult training centres

Traditionally, adult training centres were set up to provide sheltered employment for adults with learning disabilities living in the community. More recently these have become social education centres, where there is an emphasis on continuing education and the development of the skills needed to live successfully within the community. Here the speech and language clinician may work with individual clients and groups of clients and may also be involved with staff development and training. The client's time at the centre may be integrated with a range of other activities in the community, including part-time attendance at a college and work experience. Any intervention will need to be carefully coordinated and based on the current and future needs of the client.

Clients with mental health problems

Social Services departments may coordinate a range of services for people with mental health problems. They will harness resources provided by statutory agencies, and the voluntary and private sectors. Reforms in the early 1990s set out to see more services being contracted out by Social Service departments to the voluntary and private sectors.

Care coordination is a process to ensure that individual needs are met and services properly coordinated.

Children

The Children Act 1989 outlines the provision that should be made for the care of children. Although in exceptional circumstances a court order can be made to take the child into residential care, wherever possible every effort is made to keep the child in the family home. The Act states that a decision to remove the child from the home must be made only if it is in the best interests of the child. Links should be maintained with the family if at all possible.

Looked-after children

Social Services will provide residential care in the following circumstances:

- *Foster homes*: if possible the child will be placed within a family network of specially recruited and trained foster parents. They will have undergone a careful selection process and will be supported by a social work team. They will be involved with all aspects of the child's life and will be encouraged to build links with the child's natural family. They will also be responsible for keeping medical appointments and will be encouraged to work closely with all professionals involved with the child.

- *Respite care*: this may be provided for children with disabilities which may cause strain on the family. Respite care for a night, weekend or short break may be provided by specially recruited respite foster parents or through a staffed hostel. The speech and language clinician may need to give advice and training to respite carers to ensure a consistent approach to the development of communication and feeding skills.
- *Group homes*: these provide secure accommodation for children whose behaviour has made it difficult for them to remain within the family home. Specially trained staff will develop programmes and provide appropriate supervision.

Day care

- *Family centres/day nurseries*: these centres provide support for families of pre-school children. They may provide nursery care for children from the age of 3 months onwards, but will also support and work with parents. Some nursery places will be made available for children who require Social Services supervision because of suspected abuse or neglect, and others may provide special facilities for children with disabilities. The centre will be managed by a qualified nursery nurse or teacher and will be staffed by qualified nursery nurses. Some centres may also run after-school clubs. In some areas the speech and language clinician may work within the nursery setting on a regular basis. Staff may be willing to carry out programmes left by the speech and language clinician or help with running language groups or sessions with parents.
- *Play schemes*: many local authorities will run play schemes in the school holidays to provide a safe and stimulating environment for children. Special play schemes may be organized for children with disabilities.

Casework

As well as a range of day and residential services, Social Services departments will have staff who will be involved with clients on an individual basis. The casework social worker may be involved with:

- visiting families of children at risk of abuse/neglect
- supervision of children protected by a court order
- supervision of children for adoption and fostering
- statutory duties in relation to people with a mental illness who require compulsory care or compulsory hospitalization
- support and advice to all client groups and their carers
- specialist services, e.g. to blind or deaf individuals, etc.
- provision of a hospital social work service.

The speech and language clinician may need to liaise directly with an individual social worker about the needs of a client, e.g. in relation to discharge from hospital, financial hardship, etc. At other times she may be involved in a more formal way, such as in relation to child protection. Here she may be part of a large team of professionals involved with a particular child and his or her family.

Personnel

Care manager

She or he is not involved in direct service delivery but will arrange for the client to have an assessment of need. The care manager is then responsible for the design, implementation and monitoring of care to meet this need.

Care assistant

She or he may perform a range of tasks to enable the client to remain in the home environment.

Key worker

She or he usually carries the main service-providing role and is responsible for coordinating the involvement of all professionals working with the client. The key worker provides a central point for communication.

Case worker

She or he will be appointed to a client or family to give support and advice.

Occupational therapist

Some occupational therapists are employed by Social Services departments. They play an important role in the assessment and support of people with a disability, and will be involved in the provision of special equipment, adaptation to housing, etc.

Specialist social worker

Some departments will employ social workers who have specialist knowledge in relation to particular client groups, e.g. deaf people and clients with visual impairment.

Duty social worker

Social Services departments will always have a member of staff on call in an emergency. This duty social worker may deal with a crisis and then hand the client on to other staff in the department.

The voluntary and private sector

There is an increasing number of voluntary and private institutions and agencies providing health and social care to clients. Recent reorganization of Social Services provision has encouraged a range of agencies to be involved in contributing to a package of care.

Working with volunteers and in voluntary agencies

The speech and language clinician may also be involved with training and supervising volunteers in the work setting where they may be an extremely valuable resource. However, there are other issues that need to be considered.

Volunteers should be recruited only after approval from a line manager and there will usually be a Trust policy outlining the process. There should be a careful system of selection and screening of potential volunteers. It is important to check the procedures with your own personnel department because there are likely to be insurance implications, and there will be a requirement for Criminal Records Bureaux (CRB) checks and health checks to be carried out. It is also important that the role and contribution of the volunteer are clearly defined before the start of his or her involvement, and that the work is supervised closely. Clients should be consulted about the volunteer's role, and consent to his or her involvement should be gained. Some of the differences between an assistant employed by the department and a volunteer are given in Table 6.4.

Table 6.4 Some differences between an assistant and a volunteer

Assistant	Volunteer
Full-/part-time involved in range of aspects of therapy	Usually involved with one client-specific task
Obliged to keep records	No compulsion to keep records
Formal supervision essential	May not receive regular supervision
Work usually in formal setting – clinic, school, hospital	May work in clinic, hospital, school and client's home
Has job description, standards, disciplinary procedures	Has negotiated role, choice and freedom

Personnel responsible for:
  health checks
  police checks, etc.
	Needs careful vetting for:
	  health checks
	  police checks, etc.

Charitable organizations

Several charitable organizations employ their own speech and language clinicians. These agencies are usually involved in the provision of specialist care and advice for a particular client group, e.g.:

- SCOPE provides information, assessment and educational and social care for children and adults with cerebral palsy.
- Action for Dysphasic Adults (ADA) provides an information and advice service for speech and language clinicians, relatives of people with aphasia and others involved in their care.
- The Motor Neurone Disease Association provides specialist advice and support to people with motor neuron disease and their families.
- I-CAN is responsible for several residential schools for children with specific language impairment.

There are certain advantages for the clinician working in these types of settings. Probably the most important is the chance to gain specialist experience with a particular client group, and the opportunity to work alongside staff who are specialists in the field. There may also be a significantly reduced caseload in comparison with clinicians working for a statutory agency. In some instances these charities may have greater resources for equipment and additional staff training, but certainly this is not always the case.

On the other hand, in a small organization there may be little opportunity for contact with other speech and language clinicians. The management structure may mean that supervision is provided by someone from a different clinical background, who may not fully understand the role of the speech and language clinician. There are also issues such as pay, conditions and pension arrangements that may differ from employment terms with a statutory organization. Advantages include:

- experience with a specialist client group, often with specialist support
- increased autonomy and the possibility to shape your own role
- a smaller caseload
- improved resources and access to training.

Disadvantages include:

- professional isolation, because of small number employed
- isolation from broader speech and language context and developments
- organizational structure which may mean that the manager is not a speech and language clinician
- lack of recognition of experience when returning to more traditional employment
- differences in conditions of service, e.g. superannuation, holiday entitlement, etc.

The private sector

Private health care and private hospitals

In the UK, speech and language therapy is frequently not covered by private medical insurance. The provision of therapy services in private hospitals and care homes is usually on an individual basis and provided by a speech and language clinician in private practice.

Independent practice

There has been a steady increase in the numbers of speech and language clinicians being employed in the private sector or choosing to be independent practitioners. The RCSLT recommends that clinicians should have a minimum of 2 years' experience before venturing into private practice. There is now an Association of Speech and Language Therapists in Independent Practice (ASLTIIP) which is affiliated to the RCSLT. Together they have produced guidelines for liaison between clinicians employed within the NHS and therapists within the private sector (RCSLT 2003a), including the following:

- The primacy of client care usually rests with the NHS therapist if care is being shared with an independent practitioner.
- The lead role in coordination of care normally rests with the NHS therapist.
- If a client opts for private therapy while on a waiting list for NHS treatment, his or her name should remain on the waiting list unless the client specifically asks for its removal.
- An NHS therapist should not disclose any information to a private therapist without the written consent of the client/carer involved.

For further information see RCSLT (1996).

Anybody interested in working in the private sector in the UK must be registered as a private practitioner with the RCSLT and should contact ASLTIIP for advice. Clients enquiring about private therapy should be encouraged to discuss this with their GP or to contact ASLTIIP. A speech and language therapist employed by a statutory agency should not provide private therapy for any of the clients on her or his caseload. They should provide the client with information about how to contact a suitably qualified therapist.

Locum agencies

There is an increasing number of locum agencies prepared to put speech and language clinicians on their books. Although some of them will consider including newly qualified therapists on their list, it is recommended that the clinician should have had some generalized experience and have gained full clinical autonomy in a supervised setting.

These agencies may be contacted by statutory bodies or charitable/private institutions that wish to fill employment gaps. The agency will provide potential employers with details of their charges and information about of a number of clinicians who may fit the job criteria. The employer will want up-to-date information about experience, along with references from past employers and other agency experience. Any contract is likely to be short term because this is an expensive way for employers to fill vacancies.

Conclusion

The newly qualified clinician will be expected to fulfil a variety of roles in a wide range of settings, and to interact with a large number of professionals. It will be essential that she receives managerial and clinical support to ensure that her time is appropriately targeted and that the demands made on her are realistic. Mentoring, supervision and support will be essential. There are many avenues for this professional support and advice. Some of this will be through formalized networks, but much can also be gained through less formal means. Being open to the suggestions of others and listening to discussions that take place in the department will provide invaluable information. The clinician should also realize the importance of the support and information that she can bring to the department and be prepared to express her own views and discuss her own experiences.

Chapter 7
Record keeping and reporting

One of the cries heard from some clinicians is 'If only there were not so much paperwork . . . all these records, reports, letters, statements and statistics . . . it keeps me away from the real work'.

Let us think this through in a more positive way. We should never under-estimate how much written communications, records and data collection are a part of the real work. The paperwork, i.e. the information systems of records and reports, is a very significant aspect of client management and the provision of an effective and efficient service.

- Without records and reports, where is the accurate documentation of our knowledge of the client, the assessments that we have used, the intervention that we have given, the contacts with and contributions of other personnel, the responses of the client and the progress that has taken place?
- Without records and reports, how do other personnel know precisely what has taken place or become familiar with what the service provides?
- Without records and reports, how can the work of the speech and language service be objectively evaluated for effectiveness and resource needs?

Recording and reporting must be viewed not as arduous or unnecessary evils, but as integral to the delivery of speech and language services to clients, and must be respected for the role that they have in providing a formal mechanism for speech and language professional accountability.

This chapter looks in particular at three forms of information systems that have a significant place in speech and language therapy clinical practice: case records, reports and statistics. The following are the aims:

1. To provide an understanding of the purposes of information systems.
2. To consider some of the legal and ethical implications of information systems.
3. To offer guidelines for good practice in the compilation of information systems.

Case records

Case records constitute a formal record of information pertinent to the speech and language management of a particular client. As a speech and language clinician you are responsible for any entry that you have made and hence legally and professionally accountable for what is written. A speech and language case record will be kept for each client from the date of referral and retained even after discharge. This may be part of a unified health record where all health professionals record information. This helps to establish a coordinated approach to care and the sharing of good practice, but can cause difficulty getting quick access to information in a file that is being used by a fellow professional. In some cases, a separate speech and language therapy file may be maintained. However, the introduction of electronic health records by December 2005 should make this sharing of information easier. Dependent on the clinical context you may need to contribute with a range of personnel to other types of case records. Two examples of these, medical records and care plans, are explained below, in addition to the discussion of speech and language case records.

Medical records

For clients who are hospital inpatients the medical records kept on the ward are key in communications between the professionals involved, and facilitate the day-to-day multidisciplinary coordination of information about contacts made, assessment findings, diagnosis, intervention, progress and recommendations. Entries in the notes by the speech and language clinician are a professional obligation. These must be relevant and brief, respecting that no one has time to read more than the bare essentials and remembering that communication about the client is not restricted to the highlights that you include here. You will also be using other communication channels, such as ward rounds, case conferences and meetings with specific professionals, as well as written reports and regular entries in the ward Cardex system, to share information and guide the decision-making process.

In the medical records very few words can be used, e.g.:

1. To confirm that you have responded to a referral, made an initial contact, identified significant problems or an initial diagnosis, and to indicate your immediate intentions and recommendations:
   Drowsy, confused; language comprehension severely impaired; speech output restricted to unintelligible jargon; motor skills unaffected in feeding and speech. To further assess. (Your signature and the date)
2. To give information about change, family contact and advice given, and indicate future plans:
   Depressed, deterioration in swallowing function, speech no longer a viable means of communication. Patient and wife advised on alternative communication methods. Appointment with Communication Aids Centre

arranged. To continue to see after imminent discharge home. (Your signature and the date)

Care plans

This is commonly a care management plan, which is a contract of care provision that enables the delivery of a coordinated package of care for a person. Care plans might be used for a child or an adult with multiple disabilities or learning difficulties, who has a range of identified needs. This statement of needs places care within a functional and social context. A care plan might be drawn up for a person living either in his or her own or family home, or in a care home. In either case the individual may or may not attend a rehabilitation or development unit, or a day or education centre. Initially, a functional assessment of the needs of the individual would be made. Then the multidisciplinary team, together with the client and, where appropriate, his or her next of kin, guardian or advocate, would negotiate a care management plan, which specifies objectives for care and identifies the personnel responsible for providing appropriate support to meet these objectives. In this way, qualified and unqualified personnel from a range of health and social care agencies (e.g. physiotherapists, home care assistants, residential care assistants, district nurses, nursing assistants, occupational therapists, social workers, and speech and language therapists) have a common point of reference, enabling them to record and share understandings about the physical, functional and social needs of the individual, and determine the extent to which the objectives of the care management plan have been met.

Communication is one of the categories that may be included in the care plan, and for which the speech and language clinician may have direct or indirect responsibility. If this is the case, the clinician would negotiate and agree specific objectives relating to speech and language and swallowing function, record progress and recommend any modifications required in the light of change. Once more we have an information system that contains a record of evidence from a range of personnel involved in the care of the client, which will be readily available to everyone. To be effective in contributing to the care of the individual, all entries must be concise and written in language that will be accessible to everyone, including professionals from a range of disciplines and non-professional caregivers. In addition, as with any other record, entries must be dated and signed, and hence owned by the author.

Figure 7.1 gives an example of an extract from a care plan showing how the speech and language clinician contributes to the record.

Speech and language case records

The speech and language case record constitutes a file of all the data relating to the client who has been referred to the speech and language clinician. This is not merely a device to remind us about the client from week to week, but a

---

(date)
1. To locate 4 additional Blissymbols on request – garden, bird, flower, tree.
2. To spontaneously use symbols in social speech – e.g. hello, fine, hungry.
3. To initiate 2 symbol questions – e.g. where nurse? when mum (coming)? what weather (like)?

Recommendations:
    Practise location of new and previously introduced symbols.
    Engage him in social speech question and answer.
    Encourage him to ask you questions.
    (your signature)

Figure 7.1 How the speech and language clinician contributes to the record.

comprehensive account that will be passed on to other speech and language clinicians who may be involved at a later date. It is also the account that serves as the reference point for any issues relating to the case that arise during the current episode of care or in the future, even after discharge from speech and language intervention, and up to the death of the client. Hence, it is vital that as new information is known it is recorded. Even if you think that you can remember, the details will fade or distort over time, and they will not have been made available to others unless they are written down as soon as possible.

The contents of the case record file will vary. In the case of a person who was seen for initial assessment only, there may be little more than the essential client details, a minimal note of referral and background information, the assessment findings and conclusions from the meeting with the client, and a copy of the discharge report. Another person might have a more long-standing and complex history of contact with speech and language clinicians, which could result in a rather weighty case record. Further, each speech and language service will have a different framework for the record. None the less it is helpful to outline the components that will normally be included in the case record:

- client identification data
- diagnosis
- background details
- presenting problems
- intervention.

Client identification data

These includes name, date of birth, gender, address, telephone number, hospital number (if applicable), referring agent details, date of referral, GP details, school (if applicable) and next of kin. It is important also to make a note of the reason for referral, the date of the initial appointment and, when the time arrives, the date of discharge, with a note of the reason for discharge (e.g. death, transfer to another authority, mutual agreement with the client or non-attendance). Some of this information may be translated into codes for data collection and analysis (see Statistics below).

Therefore, clinicians should have all the data that they need to identify each client both in their written communications and for statistical records, and to facilitate their basic communications with and about the client.

Diagnosis

This constitutes the speech and language diagnosis made by you, the expert in speech and language pathology, e.g. 'delayed phonological disorder', 'semantic–pragmatic disorder', 'verbal dyspraxia'. In addition, it is often helpful to include a reference to any medical diagnosis and significant aetiological factors that explain the nature of the disorder, e.g. 'hearing impairment', 'auditory attention deficit', 'cerebral vascular accident', 'no known causation'.

The final diagnosis of the communication disorder may be difficult to ascertain until some time has passed and a full picture of the problem(s) has evolved from the data collection, hypothesis formulation and hypothesis testing process of assessment. Only when this point is reached are you in a position to confirm a diagnosis. However, you do need to provide at least a broad and tentative diagnosis at an early stage for the purposes of communication and statistical records. Hence, it is not uncommon for the case file to have two headings: 'Provisional diagnosis', to be completed at first contact, and 'Diagnosis', to be completed as soon as a differential diagnosis of the communication disorder has been made. Thus the provisional diagnoses of 'non-fluency', 'moderate dysarthria' and 'speech disorder', which describe three different individuals after the first contact, may be rewritten in the course of time as diagnoses of 'severe stammering', 'moderately severe progressive mixed spastic and flaccid dysarthria (caused by motor neurone disease)' and 'developmental expressive language and articulatory disorder (caused by cleft palate)'.

Background details

This includes all the case history details, as well as additional information about the client that will emerge in the course of contact with him or her. The client's background will be learned from a range of data-collection procedures, discussed in Chapter 3 (e.g. case history taken from the client and/or carer; medical notes; school reports; ongoing information from the client, family, friends and other carers and personnel who are in contact with the client). When recording information in the file, it is important to provide dates to ensure that there is a chronological record of events. In addition, you should note sources of information whenever possible so that discrepancies can be identified and evaluated, e.g. a mother might report that her child had normal hearing, but an audiogram might indicate a reduction in acuity in certain frequencies that would be of minimal concern for most children, but for a child with delayed speech and language development this may be significant.

Case files generally contain sections for key aspects of background details within which we can add information as it emerges. 'Medical', 'Personal and social' and 'Development' are common headings; however, these will obviously differ depending on the client group. The sections are likely to be guided according to the varying information that we need to record for acquired, adult, developmental or child disorders.

Presenting problems

It is always important to have a record of the disorder as it presented at the first contact with a speech and language clinician. This serves as the baseline for your future investigations and as a reference point for your evaluation of progress. Clinicians should record a description of the presenting features of the impairment, indicating the strengths, weaknesses and influences on communication function that they observe, e.g.

- Gait unsteady, clinging to mother for most of session, unable to complete simple form board; responded to name, able to identify familiar pictured items from name; follows two idea commands 50%; speech restricted to monosyllabic utterances not identifiable as words, consonants fronted.
- Good concentration and insight into communication difficulty; anxious that will be unable to return to previous employment.
  Comprehension 100% in social level conversation.
  Western Aphasia Battery: auditory verbal comprehension – 57/60, yes/no questions – 60/60, auditory word recognition/sequential commands – 70/80. Reading comprehension delayed but accurate at level of short simple paragraph. Speech output non-fluent where increased demand for specific content. Word-retrieval problems characterized by semantic paraphasia and repair, aided by phonemic cues and semantic associations. Agrammatic as a result of limited use of function words and appropriate word endings. Moderate intelligibility; able to communicate messages with some success but linguistic accuracy impaired. Spontaneous writing from picture stimulus not possible. Writing to dictation of common words legible, but only accurate in spelling simple short words with regular spellings.

Intervention

This will include a record of dates and findings of formal and informal assessments, copies of which (e.g. samples of speech, drawings and writing, as well as completed assessment record sheets from published or clinician-designed assessments) may be included as an appendix to the case file to provide evidence of performance and progress. In addition, this will contain a record of direct and indirect intervention, written in a clear but very concise style, making sure that the objectives and outcomes are identified. Where evidence is available, such as letters and reports to and from other professionals, these should also be included in chronological order in a separate section of the file.

The main body of the case record or file will be in the form of chronologically dated and signed entries. These may consist of a record of a telephone call made or received about the client, the key points of a conversation with a teacher or a summary of a session with the client. In addition, objective-based management decisions and recommendations as well as evidence of change will be noted at relevant places within the ongoing account.

It is not uncommon to have concerns about the style and acceptable content when making entries in the case file. Although each clinician will develop a somewhat idiosyncratic manner, there are golden rules that must be followed in order to meet your legal and professional obligations. The account should be:

- Accurate
- Comprehensive
- Contemporaneous, i.e. written as soon as possible after the contact; anything more than 24 hours after the event has reduced validity and credibility
- Legible – mistakes should be deleted with a signal score; erasers and correction fluid should not be used
- Relevant
- Signed and dated.

If you have planned your intervention thoroughly with clearly defined objectives, the account should be quite easy to write:

1. Remember to use unambiguous, concise language.
2. Do not use abbreviations or acronyms unless a key is also provided.
3. Indicate assessment findings and the objective for each aspect of therapy and the outcomes achieved by the client.
4. Note any observations or additional information that emerged during the contact.
5. State both the action you have taken and the recommendations you propose.
6. Date and sign the entry.

Below are two examples, one of good and one of bad practice, of case report entries written after a session with a 4-year-old boy with severe language comprehension problems:

1. Jamie arrived in a new jersey today, played happily with the cars but could not indicate the colours when asked. Would sometimes not give me the toys in the order I requested. Did not say very much today. Looked unhappy but would not say what was wrong. Apparently has been in trouble at the nursery this morning. I asked Mrs P if I could see Jamie at home next week, which she agreed.

2. Small toy play age appropriate.

   Colour concept (red and blue) development: (a) cars sorted by colour (red/blue) 100%; (b) auditory verbal comprehension of colour names 20%; (c) imitation of the colour name for the red items sorted encouraged to develop word association, achieved for all items.

   Auditory verbal memory: identification of familiar monosyllabic nouns (spoon, doll, car and ball) by name 100%. Memory for the nouns 100% for two items, 70% correct for three items and 30% for four items.

   Reserved behaviour with episodes of lapses in attention. Did not initiate conversation.

   Mother reports his difficulty in following instructions at nursery, and slowness to respond results in the other children teasing him. Agreed to contact nursery.

   Home visit arranged for next week to evaluate communication in familiar environment.

   (Signed and dated)

You can see from the second example that:
- there is no need to include the name of the child, or to mention yourself; this can be taken as known
- subjective comments (e.g. 'looks', 'seems', 'appears') must be avoided; only facts are of interest
- wherever possible, measurements should be included; from this, performance and change can be accurately conveyed
- management decisions should be clearly indicated.
- entries must be signed and dated.

A well-written entry will (RCSLT 1996):
- facilitate the delivery of service to the client
- provide documentary evidence of the service delivered
- facilitate the continuity of care
- discharge a contractual duty to the employer
- contribute to the preparation of reports and statements
- assist the mechanism of accountability
- contribute to the evaluation of the service offered.

It can also be useful to provide a summary of proposed actions, so that the clinician can quickly check that she has completed all aspects of her plan before the next meeting, e.g.

Action:
- Letter to GP regarding medication
- Phone transport to check next appointment
- Book video camera for next appointment.

Defensible documentation

Although the professional and legal status of the case records has been emphasized, this should be explained in context and with further detail to support the clinician in recording information.

The case record is a defensible document. This means that it constitutes primary evidence, i.e. original documentation, and as such can be used in litigation cases. A demand for the submission of case records for use as evidence may be made in rare instances when the management of a client by the speech and language therapy service has been questioned. More commonly, the records are required to contribute to cases of alleged medical negligence, compensation agreements, or in family or criminal cases in which the communication disorder is perceived to be a factor. This provides a further reason for the requirement to retain any record that is written during the life of an individual. Even if a record is damaged, whether by tearing or tea spillage, for legal purposes it must be retained in this state.

Professional opinion expressed on any personal health records, and this includes speech and language therapy records, remains the property of the author. It is essential to confirm authorship at the time of writing by adding the date and your normal signature, not merely by initialling the account. You should be confident that what is written is accurate, unambiguous, sufficiently detailed and legible. The author is responsible for whatever is written and so has to be prepared to defend the account if required.

As clinicians have such responsibility for what they write, they must ensure that there is no doubt about the detail and authenticity of what is included, and that it will stand up in court if necessary. First, anything written should not be altered by obliterating the original entry. Instead, you must put a single line through the error and date and initial the change. Second, if abbreviations are used, make sure that a key is supplied so that they can be understood by other personnel.

In Britain, since the Access to Health Records Act 1990, clients have had a right to access all personal information held on both manual (written) and computerized health records. The proviso is that access can be withheld if the information is deemed likely to cause them or another person physical or mental harm. This is particularly the case where the records include information about another individual who might be identified if access were given. Knowing that the client can make a request and in most cases can see the records reminds us of the importance of including objective and clear details. It is considered professionally unacceptable to record trivia or pejorative remarks, but knowing that your notes can be seen outside your own tight professional circle certainly helps focus your style.

Notes should always be dated and each page must include the client's name and identifying number. Notes should be written up within 24 hours of the contact, but it is good to get into the habit of completing them as soon as possible after the event, because it becomes much harder to remember details as time passes, and the notes will then take much longer to write up.

Computer and joint records

So far, this overview of case records has concentrated on manual systems of record keeping. In recent years, with a view to a wide range of knowledge about their clients being readily available to every professional involved in their care, computerized and joint case recording systems have been introduced in some health services. This requires a dedication to confidentiality and security of passwords so that entry to the system and information held is confined to authorized personnel. In addition, practical problems may need to be overcome, e.g. having access to a computer to input data as soon as possible after contact or other intervention, the technical skills of the clinician in receiving and inputting data, the ability of the system to cope with such things as phonetic symbols, and including data that have uniformity with those of other users. However, the use of computerized systems certainly increases the chance of professionals becoming conversant with each other's management decisions and makes information-sharing more open and speedy. In effect, it should contribute to improved client care.

Records of all types are also valuable sources of data for research and audit. Not only do records form an integral part of the management of the individual client, but they can contribute to wider contexts, such as the constant search for new understandings of communication disorders and their management and the endeavour to ensure that service provision is of the highest quality.

Electronic health records

The 1998 NHS IT strategy (Information for Health) set a programme for the implementation of electronic health records (EHRs), which should provide a 'paperless' system, and facilitate sharing of information between professionals. These systems are currently being piloted in a number of sites. All Trusts should be using EHRs by 2005.

Data protection and confidentiality

Employers within the NHS are under a legal duty to keep all patient information confidential, no matter how this information is stored (Data Protection Act 1998). The Caldicott Principles laid down by the NHS Executive must be followed at all times and each Trust will have a Caldicott Guardian who is responsible for ensuring safe storage of information. Issues of confidentiality can cause some difficulty for clinicians working in non-health-care settings where the legislation and attitude to confidentiality may be different, e.g. clinicians working within education may have access to information that cannot be shared with school staff. It is also important to consider how health notes are stored on non-NHS premises.

Use of email

Increasingly, electronic mail may be used to send reports, referrals or general information. It is important to be aware of trust policies that are in place to ensure that confidentiality is maintained. Consideration needs to be made about how and where this information is stored, so that it cannot be accessed by others. This correspondence should also be printed out, suitably labelled with date, client's name and reference number, and filed within the client's records.

Phone calls

A dated account of telephone conversations about clients should be recorded in the relevant notes, and confidentiality must be maintained. Information should not be given over the telephone unless you can be confident of the identity of the caller. The clinician needs to be aware of her employer's policy and working guidelines.

Outcome measures

Many speech and language therapy departments will use a system to evaluate therapy. Therapy Outcome Measures (TOM – Enderby and John 1997) provide an objective and standardized tool. This will be an important part of the client's case file. These measures help to assure quality and contribute to the development and improvement of services. The client's communication is evaluated and scored at initial assessment in terms of:

- impairment
- disability
- handicap
- well-being/distress.

A second evaluation is then carried out at defined intervals or discharge, and the scores can be compared.

Case reports

It is not uncommon for the inexperienced clinician to have concerns about report writing, such as when to send a report, what it should contain, how long and detailed it should be, the style in which it should be written and to whom copies should be sent. Most of these anxieties will become insignificant as you gain greater familiarity with the codes of practice of your own professional organization, and the standards and practices of the individual speech and language service where you are working, as you are exposed to examples of reports received or sent by other speech and language clinicians and as your experience of actual report writing increases. Here we offer a few general comments on some of the practical issues involved.

Broad guidance concerning report writing is provided by the Royal College of Speech and Language Therapists (RCSLT 1996), which identifies four types of reports defined by different stages of overall management:

1. An initial report following assessment
2. An interim report as and when necessary following referral
3. A closure report following discharge.
4. A report for specific purpose, e.g. Statement of Special Educational Need, court report, referral.

Local guidelines and the standards of practice of your speech and language therapy service are likely to provide more detailed information about when and how to report. Local templates with clearly defined headings may be available. In the case of interim reports, much will depend on your own judgement and on the requirements of other agencies. You are likely to report whether you have made a significant modification to the intervention that you are providing, e.g. from the provision of individual intensive therapy to a decision to review in 6 months, or if you have noted major change in the client, such as deterioration in performance, or if you decide to refer for other specialist opinion. A further reason for reporting would be in response to a request from another party, such as a lawyer, doctor, another professional or an education department.

The requirement for a report, whether initial, interim or closure, presents the clinician with a precious opportunity to bring together the evidence that they have accrued about a client in a structured manner and to draw a comprehensive evaluation at a particular point in time. This is then written down in an appropriate form for the recipient of the report.

To guide the composition of the report it is helpful to ask a series of questions. The answers should inform the structure, length, content and distribution of the report that is sent.

What is the purpose of the report?

The report will differ depending on whether it is only informing or also requesting the recipient to do something, e.g. requesting additional information, opinion or referral to another agent. In cases where a request is being made, it should be supported with evidence to justify the request, such as the basis for the need for a hearing test, a psychological assessment, a teacher's report or medical opinion.

If the purpose is to transfer the case to a speech and language clinician in another authority, a very detailed report would be appropriate. Similarly, a report contributing to legal and provision decisions may include details of specific assessments and treatments. Such elaboration would serve little usefulness to a recipient who requires a concise overview of the problems and functional effects of the disorder, the prognosis and proposals for future management, or basis for discharge.

What information should be included?

The report should include only what the recipient needs to know, and detail should be limited to that which is useful to him or her, and no more. The clinician must therefore be sensitive to the professional knowledge and to the current knowledge of the individual that the recipient is likely to have. You can use technical terms without detailed explanations if you know that the other specialist has an understanding similar to your own. The aim is to be concise. However, if the knowledge base differs this must be accommodated by alternative expressions that will be understood. The purpose of reporting is not to confuse or appear pompous but to provide meaningful information. Where various personnel are to receive the report, the content, language and style will have to be appropriately modified.

Further, it is not necessary to include information that is already known to the recipient. Where you have sent an earlier report, do not repeat what has already been said. An initial reminder of a previous report ('Following my report dated . . .') can help the recipient locate the reference, but then all that is required of you is to indicate new information and changes that have occurred since the original report. In addition, the recipient does not need to have information that they have documented or already shared with you repeated back to them.

There needs to be a careful balance between providing relevant and useful detail, and making reports concise, so that the content will be read.

Who should receive the report?

Initial reports must be sent to the referring agent. This may be a consultant, senior medical officer, GP, head teacher, a nursery manager, clinical psychologist or some other person. However, in the case of self-referral or carer referral the report is likely to be sent to the professional, perhaps the GP or head teacher, whom the clinician considers would be particularly pertinent in the coordination of information affecting the client. They should also be copied to the client unless they have indicated that they do not want this information. Subsequent reports should also be sent to the referrer so that they are appropriately updated regarding speech and language support and the client.

Copies of reports can be sent to any agent if it is in the client's interest for that person to be cognisant of the information included. It is important to remember the wide network of professionals that should be kept informed, e.g. for clients seen in hospital, a copy of the report to a consultant may be forwarded to the social worker who is currently coordinating the care of the client outside hospital, or will be after discharge. In addition to reporting to a senior medical officer, copies should be sent to the school that is involved with a child's development on a day-to-day basis. As the person responsible for primary care of the individual, the GP should be copied in to all correspondence so that he or she has a complete picture

The NHS Plan (Department of Health or DoH 2000a) has strengthened the position of patients. From April 2004, all correspondence about an individual has to be copied to them, unless otherwise stated. Therefore, it is important to consider how information can be presented in a manner that they can understand. This may require the provision of definitions or explanations of terminology, the use of simplified language or the addition of diagrams and pictures.

In some speech and language therapy services there may also be a requirement for a speech and language therapy manager to receive all reports. In this way there is a centralized access to information on clients and a valuable source of data for monitoring and audit.

It is essential at the end of the report to include a circulation list of all personnel who will be sent a copy. In this way each knows the extent to which others involved in the care of the client are being kept informed.

Finally, a copy of the report must always be kept on file in the client's case records.

What structure should the report follow?

Broadly, the report should include the following:

- An introduction, which includes client information (name, date of birth, address, hospital number), the detail of the primary recipient and a statement of the purpose of the report.
- A central part with subsections as necessary to cover a description of the communication problem, and past (if any) and present therapy.
- A summary of conclusions, including factors influencing prognosis and recommendations for future management.

Very commonly a service will have a standard form for reports. This uniformity helps other disciplines to become familiar with our ways. With standard forms headings and subheadings are likely to cover, e.g. 'Background', 'Diagnosis', 'Receptive language', 'Expressive language', 'Treatment' and 'Summary and recommendations'. Where these headings do not best meet the needs of a particular case, other headings may be added. Even if a standard format is not common practice in a service, e.g. a letter format may be preferred, it is a still advisable to use headings.

What impression do we wish to convey?

The reputation of any service is influenced by the reports that are received by other personnel. This means that the report should be informative and sensitive to the contributions of and demands on others. The style, form and content must not be in the vein of telling others what to do. Professional respect will be best achieved by a relevant, concise, well-organized and well-written report that acknowledges a need for working with others and welcomes an exchange of specialist knowledge and skills for the benefit of the client.

Short, clear sentences which progress in an orderly manner will help the reader assimilate information. Headings should be used to guide the reader through the content of the report, and an appropriate minimum of detail should be included within each section. Remember, it may only be the final summary paragraph that the reader considers is of interest or has time to look at. Make sure that this part of the report contains the key points that you wish to make.

Finally, always check grammar and spelling. Not only are errors distracting to the reader, but also speech and language clinicians without a good command of written English will not attract respect from other disciplines.

Information systems and statistics

Information systems include all the possible methods of recording, analysing and presenting data, whether manual or automated. In any business, there are three kinds of information that are important to guide planning and decision-making. These are financial, personnel and activity, or productivity, data. Clinical data may relate to any of these functions, and may be used by the health authority to monitor supply and demand, and as a basis for future funding and planning. The wealth of data recorded in health information systems are used by countless agencies concerned with the health of the population and health-care provision, e.g.:

- it is used to cost and evaluate services
- it contributes to epidemiology, i.e. the study of patterns of disorders, treatment and outcomes
- it is a source for research and audit related to health issues and health-care practice
- it is applied in personnel planning and can help identify problems, e.g. in staffing levels and sickness
- it can reflect how local or government policies are being addressed.

Accurate, relevant and current data made available from all possible sources should increase the chance of appropriately based arguments for the management decisions that affect both health-care employees and health-care users.

Data collection by speech and language clinicians is essential to provide evidence of how the speech and language service resources are employed, and this information makes a major impact on service planning and endeavours to improve efficiency. Sometimes data are recorded manually on printed forms and submitted for central input into the computer system, or they may be recorded electronically by the individual clinician. Variations depend on the sophistication of the information system of the particular authority. Although the methods, systems and codes used by different authorities vary, in essence the data related to clinicians and their day-to-day work will consist of two types of information – that associated with their working practice and that associated with their clients. Clinician information includes:

- identification details, such as a clinician code, personal information, appointment date and subsequent employment record
- daily client and non-client activities (e.g. face-to-face contact; telephone calls relating to clients; administration, from ordering stationery to completing statistics and report writing; liaison with other professionals; training; continuing professional development; attending staff meetings), the time spent on each activity and the location; holiday leave, study leave and sickness; and travel expenses.

Client information includes:

- Identification details, such as name, date of birth, address, marital status, ethnic origin, language used, need for interpreter, referring agent, type of referral (new or re-referral), disorder category (e.g. language, fluency, voice, swallowing), education status.
- Case management information, such as date of initial contact, nature (e.g. direct, indirect, individual, group) and length of subsequent contacts, and discharge details (e.g. mutual agreement between clinician and client, failed to attend, refused treatment, death, loss of contact, assessment only, transferred out of the authority, treatment not available).

The primary purpose of coordinating information about clinicians and clients is to provide accurate, quantifiable, centralized data about the service that is readily accessible to authorized personnel and agencies. From statistical analysis of the data on activity and caseloads, the features and costs of the speech and language service can be evaluated. In turn, this evidence can inform management decisions on quality improvements that are needed in provision, e.g. to support changes in patterns of referral or to increase efficiency to make best use of clinician time. The information is not only pertinent to the service itself but is required by local strategic health authorities, and will be used in making judgements about the distribution of resources and purchasing of services across the authority. Thus, it will be made available as appropriate to other interested parties, including the local authority and education departments. In addition, it will be used to inform the national picture of health and related care provision will be collected by the Department of Health.

Conclusion

In conclusion each speech and language clinician, as an employee with a responsibility to an organization, as a professional with a responsibility to clients and as an individual concerned for fairness and effectiveness in the delivery of health care, has a duty to be thorough in record keeping and reporting.

Chapter 8
Conclusions and beginnings

The preceding chapters have laid the foundations of the professional practice of speech and language clinicians. Thought has been given to contexts of work, to relationships with clients, carers and other workers, to processes and practices of case and clinical management, and to issues of professional responsibility. With this background, and the vast amounts of theoretical and experiential learning that will be covered in the course of initial training, it is hoped that the student will gain confidence and understanding, and be ready to enter employment as a registered speech and language clinician. But what next?

What does it mean to be a newly qualified speech and language clinician? It means that you have demonstrated that you have the appropriate knowledge, skills and attitudes to take responsibility for your own caseload and your own actions, to provide clients with a high quality of care, to work effectively with teams of speech and language clinicians and other workers, and to be an ambassador for the profession. It also means a commitment to continuing professional development (CPD). Learning now begins.

The transition from student clinician to clinician

There is no longer a supervising clinician who has ultimate responsibility for the decisions made and the actions taken on behalf of clients. No longer is there a carefully controlled caseload that a supervising clinician has selected to support clinical development. The newly qualified clinician may no longer have time to conduct lengthy assessments and analyse every aspect of communication of every client who is referred. No longer can she stand apart from the wide-ranging policies and procedures governing the organization in which her clinical work resides. There is no longer a carefully organized curriculum of university and practice-based learning managed by tutors and clinicians to guide academic and professional development. Now the clinician has to learn to use her time effectively so that she can establish and maintain work networks, provide maximally effective care to maximum numbers of individuals with communication difficulties, reflect on her practice, and update her knowledge and skills to their potential.

Frightening? No, exciting and challenging. With a calm, organized approach (even if the adrenaline runs riot) and the realization that your own resources and those provided by others are at your disposal, you can achieve what is expected. The following sections outline some of the support that should be available and, if it is not, this should be negotiated with your line manager in order for you to meet the recommendations of the professional body (Royal College of Speech and Language Therapists or RCSLT 1996).

Registration

'Speech and language therapist' is a protected title, and anyone who uses it must be registered with the Health Professions Council (HPC) and meet their registration criteria. The HPC is the statutory regulatory body for the allied health professions, and is responsible for:

- setting standards of conduct performance and ethics
- setting education and training standards for the professions that they regulate
- establishing the process for approving and monitoring education programmes
- maintaining a register of all those fit to practice and who meet the standards
- dealing with registrants who fail to meet the standards.

It is also recommended that clinicians become members of the RCSLT as they will provide professional insurance and a wealth of professional information, including:

- a monthly bulletin and access to the *International Journal of Language and Communication Disorders*
- full access to the RCSLT website www.rcslt.org
- communicating quality – professional standards
- client-specific competencies
- clinical guidelines and position papers.

They also provide a wealth of professional advice through a range of clinical networks and specialist advisers. They have developed a Transitional Framework for Newly Qualified Practitioners (RCSLT 2004b) for new clinicians and their managers. This encompasses areas of competence that should be developed during the first 12 months of practice.

The clinician may also wish to join a union so that they have additional professional protection and employment support.

Pay and conditions

For clinicians employed within the NHS their pay and conditions will be decided under the *Agenda for Change* agreement (Department of Health or DoH 2005a). This consists of three strands:

- Job evaluation
- Terms and conditions
- The NHS Knowledge and Skills Framework (KSF), the basis for career and pay progression (www.e-ksf.org).

All job roles are evaluated and placed in one of nine pay bands on the basis of the knowledge, responsibility, skills and effort needed for the job. It is hoped that this will break down barriers between different professional groups and provide a clear career development path. This, combined with a harmonization of terms and conditions, aims to facilitate the development of multidisciplinary teams by ensuring comparability and fairness.

The KSF provides a structure for CPD and lifelong learning. The framework consists of 30 dimensions, which identify broad functions that are required within the NHS. Most staff will receive an annual increase in pay, from one point in a pay band to the next. However, at two defined points within the band, known as 'gateways', decisions will be made about pay progression and development.

The foundation gateway

This is within the first year after an individual is appointed to a pay band. Its purpose is to check that the individual meets the demand of his or her post, and is linked to planning for development within the foundation period.

The second gateway

This is a fixed point towards the top of the pay band, and is used to confirm the individual's application of knowledge and skills across all relevant dimensions; if the clinician passes through this gateway she will progress to the top of the pay band, as long as she continues to fulfil the KSF outline for the post.

Induction

A newly qualified member of staff should be taken carefully through information about the employing organization and the speech and language clinical service. This includes briefing about the following.

Employment issues

The clinician will need to be clear about the following: what hours she is expected to work; her entitlement for annual leave and special leave for domestic, personal and family reasons; the procedures to follow in the event of sickness; the roles and responsibilities covered by the post; and how progression will be managed.

The management arrangements of the organization and the service

The clinician needs to know whom she should contact according to the type of advice or agreements that she is seeking, and to whom she is accountable and can look for support, e.g. who to contact with requests for leave, or for information about professional development opportunities, discussion of ideas about potential service improvements, requests for engaging in research, advice on conflict at work and advice about specialist areas.

Supervision, mentoring and appraisal

All clinicians should have regular supervision opportunities. The system should be established during the induction period (see below).

The policies and procedures operating in the organization and the service

The clinician needs to be familiar with the organization and service mission statements. These are the declaration of the purpose of the service and what it expects of staff in terms of professional responsibility. It is important that the clinician is made aware of health and safety issues that affect her at work, e.g. she will need to know what to do in the event of exposure to challenging behaviour or infection, what hazards to be aware of and how these should be reported, how to protect confidentiality and what guidance is in place to ensure personal safety best. All staff have a duty to assess the risks to clients, other professionals and themselves (risk assessment). This assessment may relate to risk associated with the client or their environment:

> Risk management is about reducing the likelihood of errors. Its particular aims are to reduce errors that are costly in terms of damage, discomfort, disability or distress to an individual or to limit financial loss to an organisation.
>
> Moss (1995, p. 37)

As a speech and language clinician, you also need to know about policies and procedures covering, for example, child protection, abuse of vulnerable adults, alcohol and drug use, equal opportunities, staff transport and allowances, ordering equipment, complaints and referral. Further, you need to be advised and trained in the data collection procedures that apply to the speech and language therapy service.

Commonly, the newly appointed clinician will be allowed some time to meet people, orient herself to the locality in which she is working, review the caseload and gradually build up a workload. Often the demands from others and her own enthusiasm and concern to demonstrate professional capabilities can lead to overload and stress. As a newly qualified clinician, she may feel that she is less effective than she wishes. An early lesson is to be realistic about what can be achieved. Her mentor, supervisor and line manager will all help to establish what is appropriate and acceptable.

Mentoring

Mentoring is generally put in place for newly qualified staff, and also for those returning to work after a career break and for staff taking on a new specialist role. It can operate in various ways. In general, a mentor is a more senior colleague, but not the line manager. Mentoring can take place through meetings with peers as well as the mentor. It aims to enable the individual to work through concerns, clarify understanding of policies and procedures, question and reflect on practice, learn from others, and have her development monitored, and so progress towards fuller clinical autonomy.

Rotation, shadowing, working with peers and other workplace learning

More than anywhere else, professional development occurs within the daily work of the clinician. Every day the clinician will reflect on what she does, formulate hypotheses about how to improve practice, and try out and evaluate different ways of working. Practice does not make perfect, it provides opportunities for continual reflection and change. A clinician should constantly seek new learning and ways to develop. A good clinician is a questioning clinician.

In some services there are arrangements for new staff to be employed on a rotational basis. Thus, a clinician might work for 4 months in a health clinic setting, 4 months in a hospital setting and 4 months in a school or nursery setting. This provides opportunities to build on the grounding of clinical experience with a variety of client groups gained as an undergraduate, but with the authority and freedom in decision-making of a qualified member of staff. It also allows the new clinician to become familiar with personnel, facilities and practices across the service, and gives time to define work and career preferences. It will provide a foundation for negotiations with the manager to establish how service needs and the personal and professional aspirations of the clinician can best be met.

As a student clinician, you will have found it extremely valuable to shadow and observe how experienced clinicians spend their time and how they relate to clients and other people within the scope of their work. In this context you can learn so much without having to take responsibility for the activities involved. As a new clinician, or when learning a new specialism, you will find shadowing will once again provide a very welcome and rich opportunity for learning. Shadowing not only requires carefully structured observation, but also time to discuss and reflect on what was observed. In addition, it should involve time researching the literature on related theory and practice.

Throughout her career, the clinician will benefit from shadowing more experienced clinicians, those who practise different approaches, or those with specialist expertise. This is an excellent way to learn. Some speech and language clinical services with a highly specialist department (e.g. in cleft palate, dysphagia or voice disorder) may take this even further. They may offer opportunities for staff from other authorities to spend time in shadowing and other activity in a training programme, with a view to developing similar specialist services on returning to their home authority. Obviously, while the clinician is away there will be costs to her own organization for such development opportunities. However, the absence of one clinician can provide an opening for another person to experience a new area of work if they take on the vacant position on a temporary basis. We all become stale if we remain in the same role too long. Even a short break can refresh the clinician, and variety will bring different experiences that can stimulate reflection and change, whether moving on or back to post.

Another invaluable opportunity for learning with and from others is by working alongside another speech and language clinician, e.g. running a group. From the model of the techniques, ideas and behaviours applied by the other professional, particularly if followed up by discussion, the newly qualified clinician can see new and different ways of working, reflect on her own current practices and modify her approach to the advantage of clients. Clinicians must be constantly open to improvement and change.

Time management

Clinical work requires balancing a range of demands and responsibilities and the tight deadlines that accompany them. For a new clinician it can be daunting to decide just how long to spend on a particular activity, and which activities and which people should wait, or not be involved in a schedule of work. With experience, the clinician will learn how long certain aspects of work will take, and she will learn to do things more quickly and more efficiently. She will not be so stressed if things are left undone if she is confident that her priorities were correct. There will never be sufficient resources to do everything that needs to be done. The educational experience teaches the ideals of how to be thorough, but, in practice, thoroughness has to be weighed against the demands of waiting lists, throughput, attendance at meetings, giving talks, a commitment to administration, and personal and professional development. Time constraints often mean that only what is essential can be done. Sometimes the clinician will not be able to do what would be interesting, that extra in-depth assessment or long counselling session, if it means that other clients have to be neglected. Most experienced clinicians have a personal strategy of time management. It may be helpful to work through issues of time management with a mentor or peers, or to negotiate specific staff development, perhaps an in-service training course, in this field.

Clinical supervision (non-managerial supervision)

The aim of clinical supervision is to maximize clinical effectiveness through reflective practice. Although mentoring enables the new clinician, returner or new specialist to reflect, learn and be guided through a particular stage of professional development, clinical supervision is applicable outside such stages. It is relevant throughout the career of the professional. Regular clinical supervision should be incorporated within the workload of every member of staff.

Clinical supervision will usually be with a fellow speech and language professional. This may be with a professional line manager, specialist clinician or peer. The supervisor and supervisee will negotiate a contract, which provides the ground rules for the supervision. This may cover the timing and duration, place, type, method of recording, skills and techniques, confidentiality, structure of sessions and emergency strategies (e.g. whether contact outside agreed sessions is acceptable). Clinical supervision should not be confused with counselling, although some of the techniques used by counsellors, such as listening, exploration and reflection, may be used in interactions between the supervisor and the person being supervised. Clinical supervision is distinct from the relationship with a manager. It does not involve directing or monitoring the work of the clinician. Instead, it is a forum for open discussion, based on trust and confidentiality, that provides professional support. It enables the clinician to focus on work-related difficulties, challenge coping strategies, reflect on practice and explore ways to improve service delivery, as well as celebrate success. It can help clinicians to use resources more successfully, manage workloads more effectively and improve practice, and it can reduce the chances of burnout. Clinical supervision thus contributes to the process of continual learning and personal and professional development. Supervision sessions should be documented as part of the clinician's portfolio of CPD.

Managerial supervision

Every speech and language clinician will have a manager to whom she is accountable. This may be a speech and language clinician or someone from a different professional background. The manager will provide guidance and direction, and will monitor the clinician's work. This person will have a concern for the needs of the service and the clients, as well as those of individual members of staff. Guidance, negotiation and decisions about work patterns and policies and procedures will be channelled through this manager. The manager will have a key role in facilitating personal and professional development and ensuring that the clinician can make a positive contribution to the service. The relationship should be supportive and conducted through both informal and formal contacts. As well as ongoing discussions about progress, formal meetings will be set out to review personal and professional development. These meetings vary in name and form within different services, e.g. individual performance review, staff development review or appraisal.

Individual performance review, staff development review, appraisal

The purpose of this meeting is for the clinician to review her development as a member of staff, and is an opportunity to:

- review her job description
- review what she has achieved since the last meeting and consider how far she has met previously agreed objectives
- review any difficulties she has experienced in carrying out her duties
- identify training and development opportunities
- discuss her aspirations and career expectations
- clarify with her manager what the service requires of her
- agree objectives and the timescale within which they should be achieved.

Continuing professional development

Continuing professional development is defined as:

> a range of learning activities through which professionals maintain and develop throughout their career to ensure that they retain their capacity to practice safely, effectively and legally within their evolving scope of practice.
> AHP Project – Demonstrating Competence through CPD – Final Report (2003, p. 3)

Responsible professionals will be highly motivated to engage in a wide range of learning opportunities in order to develop practice and improve service delivery. Reflective practice, i.e. the constant review of one's practice and the seeking of learning opportunities to increase knowledge, refine present skills and acquire new skills, and to apply these in the workplace, is vital for effective practice. We have already mentioned a variety of contexts for personal and professional development – induction, mentoring, work rotation, shadowing, peer discussion, peer working, workplace experience and training, non-managerial supervision, managerial supervision, reading and in-service training. Course and conference attendance, research activity, and interest and audit group involvement are among the many activities that can contribute to personal and professional development. Many of these activities can shape CPD for the clinician.

Re-registration with the Health Professions Council (HPC) will depend on a self-declaration of CPD activity. A proportion of registrants will have to submit written evidence for audit purposes.

The RCSLT (2004c) have provided a framework for defining and recording CPD, so that speech and language clinicians should have the relevant evidence if requested. This involves a four-stage cycle of planning (Figure 8.1).

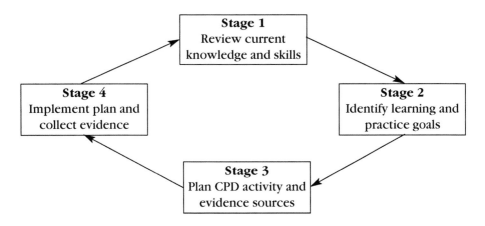

Figure 8.1 Four-stage planning for the cycle of continuing professional development (CPD).

Once learning and practice goals have been defined, usually through the appraisal or individual performance review (IPR) process, an extensive range of activities may be used to achieve these goals, which could include the following:

- **Work-based learning**: clinical audit, reflective practice, peer observation, journals club.
- **Professional activity**: membership of special interest group (SIG), mentoring, teaching, presentation at conferences.
- **Formal education**: courses, research, distance learning, planning or running a course.
- **Self-directed learning**: reading, reviewing books/articles, using the internet to update knowledge.

Although the structure for CPD is still under development, it is thought that there will be a progression of learning and career development that will link with the KSF, and the progression gateways:

Initial qualification → Unstructured CPD → Assessed CPD → Postgraduate certificate → Postgraduate diploma → Masters Degree → PhD

The RCSLT (1996) states that a full-time speech and language clinician must devote the equivalent of 10 (half-day) sessions per year to relevant continuing personal and professional development activity. It is important to recognize how much development is achieved within day-to-day work and does not have to depend solely on course or conference attendance or formal research. It is easy to establish a profile of CPD that far exceeds the minimum stated requirement for professional registration. A range of possible activities is discussed in more detail below.

Courses, workshops, seminars and conferences

A course could require anything from working towards a postgraduate degree to undertaking a non-certificated, i.e. non-assessed, course that may be only a few hours in duration. Courses may involve learning with non-speech and language clinicians. They may be offered through a variety of contexts, such as lectures, workshops or seminars, and in some instances through distance learning. They may be conducted as an in-service provision within an employing organization, or delivered by some other organization, such as another health provider, a private company or a university.

When a series of sessions is offered intensively, generally on a large scale, the term 'conference' will apply. Like many forms of courses, these offer excellent opportunities not only to learn from arranged sessions of presentations and seminars, but also from informal contacts between sessions and, particularly in residential settings, the exchanges that take place at the end of the day. It is during the informal meetings that supportive networks can be established. Conferences, and many courses, commonly provide opportunities for suppliers to display books, assessments, therapy materials and information leaflets relevant to the specialist area(s) covered, and hence are a valuable source of updating.

Books, journals, articles and the internet

Reading about aspects of professional practice is an obvious way to update knowledge. The clinician should regularly read professional and specialist journals, research into specific theories and approaches when she needs more knowledge to manage an individual case, and make time to discover and read books that will inform her professional practice. The internet can be a great source of useful information, but needs to be carefully evaluated. Anyone can post information that may be located by a search engine. This information may be anecdotal and may not have been peer reviewed. The National Library for Health (www.nelh.co.uk) provides access to clinical guidelines and e-journals, and has a speech and language therapy portal. Websites hosted by recognized charities or professional bodies may also provide access to reliable information. It is important to remember that learning from reading can be enriched by discussion, and that sharing with others will both help to clarify understanding and contribute to a greater understanding across a group of colleagues. Journal clubs are sometimes developed for this purpose, quite often as an informal network, and may perhaps be held during lunchtimes. The 'club' might be restricted to speech and language clinicians, but may extend to other personnel in the workplace. Members take turns to talk about interesting research papers as a starting point for group discussion. This means that clinicians are exposed to ideas and practices on which they may not have otherwise focused, which may stimulate new approaches in their work.

It is often from the combination of an enquiring mind, clinical experience and the opportunity to read and discuss with other colleagues that the seeds are sown for active research.

Research

The possibility that the clinician will become involved in formal research at some time or other in her career is today greater than ever. The value of evidence-based practice and a scientific investigation of theory and practice are now well recognized for both informing clinical practice and the professional development of practitioners. The evidence base for many aspects of speech and language intervention is still in its infancy, and research contributions can seem to make such a small impact when compared with all the questions that remain unanswered. Remember that any research, however small scale, will make a contribution, and that the experience of research will itself shape the clinician's own thinking, knowledge and understanding.

Research might be conducted as an individual or in collaboration with others from the speech and language or other discipline. It might be undertaken with a view to gaining a research degree. This may be funded research, perhaps supported by monies from an employing organization or the region, or from national research award bodies. Research may be either large- or small-scale; it should be carried out with the intention of sharing the results and experience with others. This may be by presenting the work at a meeting, seminar or conference, or publishing it in a paper that will be read by fellow speech and language clinicians or other people for whom the study has relevance.

McConkey (1991) suggests that within speech and language clinical practice there are three main areas of research:

1. Client characteristics, such as:
   - descriptions of language characteristics
   - relationships of certain language patterns to certain disorder categories
   - surveys, e.g. of geographical distributions of certain disorders.
2. Effectiveness of what we do, such as:
   - pre- and post-therapy comparisons
   - comparisons of different types of therapy
   - the nature of the therapy that brought about change.
3. Service effectiveness, such as:
   - consideration of different intensities of input
   - the use of different personnel to offer input.

We have stressed throughout this text that a speech and language clinician's work with clients will be informed by a scientific approach. Every time a clinician sees a client and goes through the scientific process of investigating the nature of that client's problems, recording what she is doing and planning therapy based on what she has discovered, she is engaged in 'research'. The difference between this and the more formalized procedure of research is based mainly on, first, the systematic nature of the process and, second, the dissemination of the information. The systematic nature of the process includes the following:

- Thorough exploration and a literature search to establish a problem to be investigated, questions to be answered and/or a hypothesis to be tested.
- Conducting carefully designed subject selection and data collection procedures.
- Presenting and analysing the results.
- Drawing conclusions from the findings that will contribute to understanding and identify ways forward for the progression of related research.

The traditional philosophy behind scientific enquiry, or research, is that of positivism, the fact that knowledge can be derived only from empirical, i.e. observable, evidence, e.g. establishing the causes of a disorder from examination of case data, the features of a disorder from an analysis of a speech sample, or how people change as an outcome of intervention from testing performance. This framework informs a great deal of the research carried out by speech and language clinicians. In addition, there is a wealth of understanding that cannot be observed and measured which is equally significant in the development of professional issues and practice, e.g. we not only want to know about change resulting from intervention using quantitative measures of the test results or observed performance of clients, but also need to consider their opinion about the process through which they were taken. Thus, qualitative research that investigates the opinions, attitudes, perceptions and beliefs of individuals plays a vital role in the development of professional practice.

The dissemination of the information

We fail in our responsibility as researchers and professionals if the outcomes of the investigation are not shared with, or disseminated to, other people. Research is not only about striving for personal development, but also about striving to make a contribution to our own profession and beyond and to future research.

There are many ways of sharing work with others: the choice will be guided by the size, type and purpose of the study and the range of people to be reached. Written dissemination might be in the form of a research report or dissertation of a research degree, an article in the newsletter published by specific groups of professionals or agencies that need to be influenced, a poster at a conference or a paper in a journal. Alternatively, dissemination might be achieved through oral presentation, such as at a seminar, conference, workshop, discussion group or meeting. It is important to remember that research will require not only a commitment from the individual, but also an investment by her employer. This will have been granted only if the research is perceived to be of value to both parties. The clinician has a duty to recognize that investment by making public the outcome of that investment.

Whatever sort of researcher the clinician turns out to be, it is worth reflecting on the list of qualities summarized by McConkey (1991):

- The researcher is a questioning person, not content with the status quo.
- The researcher is creative and enjoys thinking of new approaches.
- The person who researches is a risk-taker, prepared to discover uncomfortable truths.
- As much of research is about being organized, the researcher is a good manager.
- The researcher must be diplomatic and able to negotiate with a wide range of people.
- The researcher must be numerate and happy to deal with numbers and figures.
- Finally, the researcher is a plodder, willing to keep going until the project has been completed.

The clinician may not recognize all of these qualities in herself, but she will be able to relate to some of them, and others with whom she works will probably relate to different ones. This is why research, or at least some aspects of the process, is best carried out with others, and why the clinician should always seek support, whether from a research supervisor, research coordinator, experienced researchers and statisticians, or colleagues.

Special interest groups, local groups

The benefits of learning with and from others cannot be overemphasized. To this end, there are several types of formally arranged networks or groups that the clinician may be able or even required to access. SIGs consist of clinicians who have a common specialist interest. They may be for any of the following: clinicians working in special schools or in mainstream schools; clinicians working with adults with learning disability, cleft palate, head and neck disorders, semantic–pragmatic disorders or dysphagia; or clinicians with an interest in approaches such as cognitive neuropsychology. Teams of interested clinicians in a region generally organize SIGs. However, many are organized at a national level and are recognized and supported by the RCSLT. Meetings may involve guest speakers and discussion, as well as proactive activities such as the development of information leaflets. Very often, it is difficult to decide which group to join when several relate to the range of clinical interests. Remember that involvement in groups such as this demands time, often beyond attendance at meetings, if they are to be of maximum benefit. The clinician should ensure management approval and support, and guard against over-commitment of time.

Local groups are formed by the clinicians in a local region, and the members will have a range of clinical interests, although their common objective will be to share experiences and practices and to promote the profession. Projects such as those that raise awareness about communication disability are often taken on by these groups. Similar to SIGs, the presentations arranged are often open to any interested clinician and not confined to those in the locality or with formal membership of the group.

Clinical and service governance and clinical audit

Clinical governance is:

> The system through which NHS organizations are accountable for continuously improving the quality of their services and safeguarding high standards of care, by creating an environment in which clinical excellence will flourish.
>
> DoH (2005b)

Some services prefer to use the term 'service governance' because processes should include all aspects of service provision and involve all staff, as well as service users and carers. All services within an organization will have a clinical or service governance plan that will cover activities in a range of areas, including:

- the patient experience
- use of information
- quality improvement processes

The Commission for Health Improvement (CHI) will consider these plans and the work being carried out as part of their review. In addition to the individual clinician striving for the greatest effectiveness within her own case management, audit groups are commonly set up within speech and language clinical services to enable clinicians from a defined discipline, or from across a service, jointly to evaluate or audit the outcomes of clinical activity and the structure and processes of the service. Multidisciplinary audit groups may look at the overall care of clients from one particular disorder category, e.g. stroke. In this way, best practice can be identified and change proposed and implemented after a peer group exercise. At the same time, it is an opportunity for the individual clinician to learn about the practices and experiences of others and to explore alternatives, which in turn contributes to personal and professional development. It will be helpful at this point to explain a little further about audit:

Clinical audit is a process in which doctors, nurses and other health professionals systematically review, and where necessary make changes to, the care and treatment they provide to patients.

Audit Office (1995, p. 2)

Audit enables professionals to evaluate whether the standards set for the service that they are delivering are being met. They will consider the quality of the service provided in terms of the following:

- **Effectiveness**: whether the service is achieving its objectives, e.g. providing treatment that benefits the clients.
- **Efficiency**: whether the service is cost-effective, e.g. maximizing the numbers of clients seen and the range of services provided within the budget.
- **Equity**: whether the service is fairly provided, e.g. across geographical, social or ethnic groups.
- **Appropriateness**: whether the service is relevant to the needs of the community that it serves.
- **Acceptability**: whether the activities of the service are acceptable to groups and society at large.
- **Accessibility**: whether the service is offered at times and locations that suit the community that it serves.

Audit can be carried out in many different ways. Among the many means by which audit can be conducted are: random sampling of reports to referring agents or of speech and language case records; surveys of accommodation, equipment and client satisfaction; staff appraisal or individual performance review; and peer observation, case discussion and information-sharing about clinical approaches and problems. An essential aspect of audit is that findings are recorded and evaluated and reported to managers, together with recommendations, so that action can be taken to improve service delivery. The College of Speech and Language Therapists (1993) has published a useful manual that guides clinicians who may be new to the process of audit.

Audit is yet another activity that provides the clinician with opportunities to learn, reflect and achieve personal and professional development, and at the same time contribute to the delivery of a quality service.

Conclusion

This text can provide only a taster of speech and language clinical practice. As a professional, the speech and language clinician has extensive responsibilities – to her clients, her employer, herself and her colleagues. At times, it will be daunting, at times stressful, but for the most part clinicians discover that the challenges and rewards far outweigh the anxieties. At the same time, this chapter highlights the informal and formal support systems that are always on hand, not least those provided by the network of fellow speech and language clinicians and other work colleagues. This support and a professional attitude, commitment to team working, natural empathy, individual personality and the continuing development of knowledge and skills will keep the clinician on course.

This book has attempted to provide a framework for working practices, interventions with clients, and personal and professional development. Armed with this information the speech and language clinician should be able to launch herself with confidence into clinical work.

References

Acheson T (1998) Independent Inquiry into Inequalities in Health Report. London: HMSO.

Adams C, Byers Brown B, Edwards M (1997) Developmental Disorders of Language, 2nd edn. London: Whurr.

Allen C (1992) In their own times. Nursery World 4: 12-13.

Ambrose N, Yairi E, Cox N (1993) Genetic aspects of early childhood stuttering. Journal of Speech and Hearing Research 36: 701-6.

American Speech-Language-Hearing Association and the International Association of Logopedics and Phoniatrics (1994) An International Directory of Education for Speech-Language Pathologists (Speech Therapists/Logopedists/Orthophonites). Rockville, MA: ASHA.

Andolina M (2001) Critical Thinking for Working Students. Delmar: Thompson Learning.

Atkinson M, McHanwell S (2002) Basic Medical Science for Speech and Language Therapy Students. London: Whurr.

Audit Office (1995) Press Notice 64/950 on NHS (England): Clinical Audit in England. London: Audit Office

Bannister D (1982) Knowledge of self. In: Purser H (ed.), Psychology for Speech Therapists. London: British Psychological Society, pp. 194-207.

Barker P (1998) Basic Family Therapy, 4th edn. Oxford: Blackwell

Barry C (1991) Acquired disorders of reading and spelling: a cognitive neuropsychological perspective. In: Code C (ed.), The Characteristics of Aphasia. Hove, East Sussex: Lawrence Erlbaum, pp. 178-99.

Beech J, Harding L, Hilton-Jones D (eds) (1993) Assessment in Speech and Language Therapy. London: Routledge.

Belbin M (1993) Team Roles at Work. Oxford: Butterworth Heinemann.

Bernhart B, Major E (2005) Speech, language and literacy skills 3 years later: a follow up study of early phonological and metaphonological intervention. International Journal of Language and Communication Disorders 40: 1-27.

Best W, Howard D, Bruce C, Gatehouse C (1998) A treatment for anomia combining semantics, phonology and orthography. In: Chiat S, Law J, Marshall J (eds), Language Disorders in Children and Adults. London: Whurr, pp. 102-29.

Bigland S, Speake J (1992) Semantic Links. Ponteland: STASS Publications.

Bishop DVM (1989) Test for the Reception of Grammar, 2nd edn. Manchester: Department of Psychology, University of Manchester.

Bishop DVM (1997) Uncommon Understanding: Development and disorders of language comprehension in children. Hove, East Sussex: Psychology Press.

Black M, Chiat S (2003) Linguistics for Clinicians. London: Arnold.

Bower T (1987) Special Educational Needs and Resource Management. London: Croom Helm.

Breakwell G (1990) Interviewing. London: Routledge, BPS Books.

Brechin A (1999) Understandings of learning disability. In: Swain J, French S (eds), Therapy and Learning Difficulties: Advocacy, participation and partnership. Oxford: Butterworth Heinemann, pp. 58–80.

Brechin A, Swain J (1988) Professional/client relationships: creating a working alliance with people with learning disabilities. Disability, Handicap and Society 3: 213–26.

Brumfitt S (1999) Social Psychology of Communication Impairment. London: Whurr.

Bunning K (2004) Speech and Language Therapy Intervention: Frameworks and processes. London: Whurr.

Byers Brown B, Edwards M (1989) Developmental Language Disorders. London: Whurr.

Byers Brown B, Gilbert J (1989) The profession at work. In: Leahy M (ed.), Disorders of Communication: The science of intervention. London: Taylor & Francis, pp. 53–102.

Byng S (1995) What is aphasia therapy? In: Code C, Muller D (eds), Treatment of Aphasia: From theory to practice. London: Whurr.

Byng S, Black M (1995) What makes a therapy? Some parameters of therapeutic intervention in aphasia. European Journal of Disorders of Communication 30: 303–16.

Byng S, Pound C, Parr S (2000) Living with aphasia: a framework for therapy interventions. In: Papathanasiou I (ed.), Acquired Neurogenic Communication Disorders. A clinical perspective. London: Whurr, pp. 49–75.

Chandler R, Pickering C (2004) Making the most of what you have. Bulletin 622: 10–11.

Clegg JA (1993) Putting people first: A social constructionist approach to learning disability. British Journal of Clinical Psychology 32: 389–406.

College of Speech and Language Therapists (1991) Communicating Quality: Professional Standards for Speech and Language Therapists. London: College of Speech and Language Therapists.

College of Speech and Language Therapists (1993) Audit: A Manual for Speech and Language Therapists. London: College of Speech and Language Therapists.

Cooper J, Moodley M, Reynell J (1978) Helping Language Development. London: Edward Arnold.

Costello J (1993) Behavioural treatment of stuttering children. In: Prins D, Ingham R (eds), Treatment of Stuttering in Early Childhood: Methods and issues. San Diego, CA: College-Hill Press, pp. 69–112.

Council of Local Education Authorities (1994) Letter to Jeffrey, DFE, 10 February. London: CLEA.

Crystal D (1982) Profiling Linguistic Disability. London: Edward Arnold.

Crystal D, Fletcher P, Garman M (1989) Grammatical Analysis of Language Disability, 2nd edn. London: Whurr.

Crystal D, Varley R (1998) Introduction to Language Pathology, 4th edn. London: Whurr.

Dalton P (1994) Counselling People with Communication Problems. London: Sage.

Dalton P, Dunnett G (1992) A Psychology for Living: Personal construct theory for professionals and clients. Chichester: John Wiley & Sons.

Davies P, van der Gaag A (1992) The professional competence of speech therapists: III Skills and skill mix possibilities. Clinical Rehabilitation 6: 311–24.

Davis GA, Wilcox MJ (1981) Incorporating parameters of natural conversation in aphasia treatment. In Chapey R (ed.), Language Intervention Strategies in Adult Aphasia. Baltimore, MA: Williams & Wilkins.

Davis GA. Wilcox MJ (1985) Adult Aphasia Rehabilitation: Applied pragmatics. Windsor: NFER-Nelson.

Dawkins R (1986) The Blind Watchmaker. London: Penguin.

de Bono E (1985) Tactics: The art and science of success. London: Collins.

Dean EC, Howell J (1986) Developing linguistic awareness: a theoretically based approach to phonological disorders. British Journal of Disorders of Communication 21: 223-38.

Dean EC, Howell J, Waters D, Reid J (1995) Metaphon: a metalinguistic approach to the treatment of phonological disorder in children. Clinical Linguistics and Phonetics 9: 283-321.

Department of Education and Science (1978) Warnock Report: Committee of Inquiry into the Education of Handicapped Children and Young People Special Educational Needs. London: HMSO.

Department of Education and Science (1981) Education Act. London: HMSO.

Department of Education and Science (2000) Standards Fund for 2000-2001. Circular 16/99. London: DES.

Department of Education and Science (2001) SEN Toolkit. London: DES.

Department of Education and Skills (2001) Special Educational Needs: Code of Practice. London: DfES.

Department of Education and Skills (2003) Every Child Matters. London: DfES.

Department of Education and Skills (2004) Removing Barriers to Achievement. London: DfES.

Department of Health (1993) Mental Illness: Key area handbook. London: DoH.

Department of Health (2000a) The NHS Plan: A plan for investment, a plan for reform. London: HMSO.

Department of Health (2000b) No Secrets: Guidance on developing and implementing multi-agency policies and procedures to protect vulnerable adults from abuse. London: HMSO.

Department of Health (2001a) Valuing People: A new strategy for learning disability for the 21st century. London: DoH.

Department of Health (2001b) National Service Frameworks for Older People. London: DoH (www.dh.gov.uk).

Department of Health (2004) Every Child Matters. London: DoH.

Department of Health (2005a) Agenda for Change: NHS terms and conditions of service handbook. London: HMSO.

Department of Health (2005b) Definition of clinical governance: www.doh.gov.uk

Dockerill J, Henry C (1993) Assessment of mentally handicapped individuals In: Beech J, Harding L, Hilton-Jones D (eds), Assessment in Speech and Language Therapy. London: Routledge, pp. 149-62.

Dodd B (ed.) (1995) Procedures for classification of subgroups of speech disorder. In: Differential Diagnosis and Treatment of Children with Speech Disorder. London: Whurr, pp. 49-64.

Dunn LM, Dunn LM, Whetton C, Burley J (1997) BPVS II: British Picture Vocabulary Scale, 2nd edn. Windsor: NFER-Nelson.

Dryden W (ed.) (1990) Approaches to individual therapy: some comparative reflections. Individual Therapy: A handbook. Milton Keynes: Open University Press, pp. 273-81.

Duncan D (ed.) (1989) Working with Bilingual Language Disability. London: Chapman & Hall.

Dunn LM, Dunn LM, Whetton C, Pintile D (1982) British Picture Vocabulary Scale. Windsor: NFER-Nelson.

Edwards S, Fletcher P, Garman M, Hughes A, Letts C, Sinka I (1997) The Reynell Developmental Language Scales III. Windsor: NFER-Nelson.

Egan G (1978) The Skilled Helper: A systematic approach to skilled helping. Pacific Grove, CA: Brooks Cole.

Egan G (1994) The Skilled Helper: A problem-management approach to helping, 5th edn. pacific Grove, CA: Brooks Cole.

Elks L, McLachlan H (2004) Language Builders. Elklan, PO Box 79, Bodmin, PL30 3ZX.

Ellis A, Young A (1998) Human Cognitive Neuropsychology: A textbook with readings. Hove, East Sussex: Psychology Press.

Enderby P (1992) Outcome measures in speech therapy: impairment, disability, handicap and distress. Health Trends 24(2): 61–6.

Enderby P, Emerson J (1995) Does Speech and Language Therapy Work? A review of the literature. London: Whurr.

Enderby P, John A (1997) Therapy Outcome Measures (Speech and Language Therapy). London: Singular Press.

Eysenck M (2001) Principles of Cognitive Psychology, 2nd edn. Hove, East Sussex: Psychology Press.

Fabb N (1994) Sentence Structure. London: Routledge.

Fawcus M (ed.) (1992) Group dynamics and group structure. In: Group Encounters in Speech and Language Therapy. Kibworth: Far Communications, pp. 1–6.

Ferguson A, Armstrong E (2004) Reflections on speech-language therapists' talk: implications for clinical practice and education. International Journal of Language and Communication Disorders 39: 469–507.

Fielder M (1993) FIRST Screening Test. Abergavenny: Nevill Hall Hospital.

Finkelstein V (1993) From curing or caring to defining disabled people. In: Walmsley J, Reynolds J, Shakespeare P, Woolfe R (eds), Health, Welfare and Practice: Reflecting on roles and relationships. London: Sage/Open University, pp. 139–43.

Foxen T, McBrien J (1981) Training Staff in Behavioural Methods. Trainee workbook. Manchester: Manchester University Press.

Fransella F, Dalton P (2000) Personal Construct Counselling in Action, 2nd edn. London: Sage.

Frederickson N, Frith U, Reason R (1997) Phonological Assessment Battery. Windsor: NFER-Nelson.

Gardner H (1997) Are your minimal pairs too neat? The dangers of phonemicisation in phonology therapy. European Journal of Disorders of Communication 32: 167–75.

Gibbard D (1994) Parental-based intervention with pre-school language delayed children. European Journal of Disorders of Communication 29: 131–50.

Gipps C, Gross H, Goldstein H (1987) Warnock's Eighteen Per Cent. London: The Falmer Press.

Girolametto L (1988) Developing dialogue skills: the effects of a conversational model of language intervention. In: Marfo K (ed.), Parent–Child Interaction and Developmental Disabilities. New York: Praeger, pp. 53–67.

Gorrie B, Parkinson E (1995) Phonological Awareness Procedure. Ponteland, Northumberland: STASS Publications.

Gray B, Ridden G (1999) Lifemaps of People with Learning Difficulties. London: Jessica Kingsley.

Green R (1992) Supervision as an essential part of practice. Human Communication February: 21–2.

Grunwell P (1985) Phonological Assessment of Child Speech (PACS). Windsor: NFER-Nelson.

Grunwell P (1987) Clinical Phonology, 2nd edn. London: Croom Helm.

Hall D, Elliman D (2003) Health for All Children: 4th Report. Oxford: Oxford University Press.

Hall DMB (1989) Health for All Children: A programme for child surveillance. Oxford: Open University Press.

Hargie O, Saunders C, Dickson D (1994) Social Skills in Interpersonal Communication, 3rd edn. London: Routledge.

Harley T (1995) The Psychology of Language: From data to theory. London: Taylor & Francis.

Harrow J, Shaw M (1992) The manager faces the consumer. In: Willcocks L, Harrow J (eds), Rediscovering Public Services Management. London: McGraw-Hill, pp. 113-140.

Health Professions Council (2003) Standards of Proficiency for Speech and Language Therapists (www.hpc-uk.org).

Herbert M (1981) Behavioural Treatment of Problem Children. London: Academic Press.

Heron J (1990) Helping the Client: A creative practical guide. London: Sage.

Hesketh A (2004) Early literacy achievement of children with a history of speech problems. International Journal of Language and Communication Disorders 39: 453-68.

Hickman J (2002) Issues of service delivery and auditing. In: Abudarham S, Hurd A (eds), Management of Communication Needs in People with Learning Disability. London: Whurr, pp. 1-32.

Higgs J, Jones M (eds) (2000) Clinical reasoning in the health professions. In: Clinical Reasoning in the Health Professions, 2nd edn. Oxford: Butterworth Heinemann, pp. 3-22.

Higgs J, Titchen A (2000) Knowledge and reasoning. In: Higgs J, Jones M (eds), Clinical Reasoning in the Health Professions, 2nd edn. Oxford: Butterworth Heinemann, pp. 23-32.

Howard D, Hatfield F (1987) Aphasia Therapy: Historical and contemporary issues. Hove, East Sussex: Lawrence Erlbaum.

Howell J, Dean E (1994) Treating Phonological Disorders in Children: Metaphon - theory to practice, 2nd edn. London: Whurr.

Hubbell RD (1981) Children's Language Disorders: An integrated approach. Engelwood Cliffs, NJ: Prentice-Hall.

Ingram D (1989) Phonological Disability in Children, 2nd edn. London: Whurr.

Invalid Children's Aid Nationwide (2004) Learning Together: Working Together. London: I-CAN

Isaac K (2002) Speech Pathology in Cultural and Linguistic Diversity. London: Whurr.

Jeffree D (1996) Observation of play in the early assessment and development of children with severe learning difficulties. In: Fawcus M (ed.), Children with Learning Difficulties: A collaborative approach to their education and management. London: Whurr, pp. 37-63.

Kay J, Lesser R, Colthart M (1997) PALPA: Psycholinguistic Assessment of Language Processing in Aphasia. Hove, East Sussex: Psychology Press.

Kelly G (1955/1991) The Psychology of Personal Constructs. New York: Norton. Reprinted 1991 by Routledge, London.

Kelly J, Local J (1989) Doing Phonology. Manchester: Manchester University Press.

Keresz A (1982) The Western Aphasia Battery (WAB). New York: Grune & Stratton.

Kineen L (1994) A journey towards a quality service. Journal of Clinical Speech and Language Studies 4: 45-55.

Knowles W, Masidlover M (1982) The Derbyshire Language Scheme. Education Office, Ripley, Derbyshire.

Kolb D (1994) Organizational Behavior: An experiential approach. Englewood Cliffs, NJ: Prentice Hall.

Ladefoged P (1982) A Course in Phonetics, 2nd edn. San Diego: Harcourt Brace Jovanovich.

Lahey M (1988) Language Disorders and Language Development. New York: Macmillan.

Lawson R, Pring T, Fawcus M (1993) The effects of short courses in modifying attitudes of adult and adolescent stutterers to communication. European Journal of Disorders of Communication 28: 299-308.

Leahy M (1989) The philosophy of intervention. In: Leahy M (ed.), Disorders of Communication: The science of intervention. London: Taylor & Francis, pp. 3-12.

Leahy M (1995) Self-perception: the therapist in the process of change. In: Wirz S (ed.), Perceptual Approaches to Communication Disorders. London: Whurr, pp. 131-45.

Lees J, Urwin S (1997) Children with Language Disorders, 2nd edn. London: Whurr.

Lesser R (1992) The making of logopedists: an international survey. Folia Phoniatrica 44: 105–25.

Levelt W (1989) Speaking: From intention to articulation. Cambridge, MA: MIT Press.

Lock S, Wilkinson R, Bryan K (2001) Supporting Partners of People with Aphasia in Relationships and Conversation (SPPARC). Bicester: Speechmark.

Lubinski R (1994) Environmental systems approach to adult aphasia. In: Chapey R (ed.), Language Intervention Strategies in Adult Aphasia, 3rd edn. Baltimore, MA: Williams & Wilkins, pp. 269–91.

McAllister L, Lincoln M (2004) Clinical Education in Speech-Language Pathology. London: Whurr.

McAllister L, Rose M (2000) Speech-language pathology students: Learning clinical reasoning. In: Higgs J, Jones, M (eds), Clinical Reasoning in the Health Professions, 2nd edn. Oxford: Butterworth Heinemann, pp. 205–13.

McCartney E (1999) Barriers to collaboration: an analysis of systemic barriers to collaboration between teachers and speech and language therapists. International Journal of Language and Communication Disorders 34: 431 – 440.

McConkey R (1991) Practitioners as researchers. Journal of Clinical Speech and Language Studies 1: 1–15.

McDaniel D, McKee C, Smith Cairns H (1996) Methods for Assessing Children's Syntax. Cambridge, MA: MIT Press.

McLeod J (1997) Narrative and Psychotherapy. London: Sage.

Marschark M, Siple P, Lillo-Martin D, Campbell R, Everhart V (1997) Relations of Language and Thought: The view from sign language and deaf children. Oxford: Oxford University Press.

Marshall J (1998) Introduction. In: Chiat S, Law J, Marshall J (eds), Language Disorders in Children and Adults. London: Whurr, pp. 71-6.

Marshall J, Black M, Byng S, Chiat S, Pring T (1999) The Sentence Processing Resource Pack. Bicester, Oxon: Winslow.

Martin S (1987) Working with Dysphonics. Bicester, Oxon: Winslow Press.

Miller J (1981) Assessing Language Production in Children. Baltimore, MA: University Park Press.

Miller N, Docherty G (1995) Acquired neurogenic speech disorders: applying linguistics to treatment. In: Grundy K (ed.), Linguistics in Clinical Practice, 2nd edn. London: Whurr, pp. 358–64.

Moss F (1995) Risk management and the quality of care. In: Vincent C (ed.), Clinical risk Management. London: BMA Books.

NHS Circular (1999) For the Record. Managing records in NHS Trusts and health authorities. London: HMSO.

NHS Circular (2001a) Good Practice in Consent –HSC 2001/023. London: HMSO.

NHS Circular (2001b) Seeking Consent: Working with children. London: HMSO.

Oates J, Grayson A (2004) Cognitive and Language Development in Children. Oxford: Blackwell.

Onslow M (1992) Identification of early stuttering: issues and suggested strategies. American Journal of Speech and Language Pathology 1: 21-7.

Parasuraman A, Zeithaml V, Berry L (1985) A conceptual model of service quality and its implications for future research. Journal of Marketing 19(6): 5–11.

Parker A, Irlam S (1995) Speech intelligibility and deafness: the skills of listener and speaker. In: Wirz S (ed.), Perceptual Approaches to Communication Disorders. London: Whurr, pp. 56–83.

Parker A, Kersner M (2001) Developing as a speech and language therapist. In: Kersner M, Wright J (eds), Speech and Language Therapy: The decision-making process when working with children. London: David Fulton Publishers, pp. 12-29.

Perkins M, Howard S (eds) (1995) Principles of clinical linguistics. In: Case Studies in Clinical Linguistics. London: Whurr, pp. 10-35.

Phelps-Terasaki D, Phelps-Gunn T (1992) Test of Pragmatic Language. Austin, TX: Pro-Ed.

Pound C, Parr S, Lindsay J, Woolf C (2000) Beyond Aphasia: Therapies for living with communication disability. Bicester, Oxon: Winslow Press.

Priestley P, McGuire J (1983) Learning to Help: Basic skills exercises. London: Tavistock Publications.

Prochaska J, DiClemente C (1986) Towards a comprehensive model of change. In: Miller W, Heather N (eds), Treating Addictive Behaviors. New York: Plenum Press, pp. 162-183.

Purchell M, McConkey R, Morris I (2000) Staff communication with people with intellectual disabilities: the impact of a work-based training programme. International Journal of Language and Communication Disorders 35: 147-158.

Rapp B (2001) The Handbook of Cognitive Neuropsychology: What deficits reveal about the human mind. Hove, East Sussex: Psychology Press.

Reilly S (2004) What constitutes evidence? In: Reilly S, Douglas J, Oates J (eds), Evidence-Based Practice in Speech Pathology. London: Whurr, pp. 18-34.

Renfrew C (2001) The Renfrew Language Scales. Bicester: Speechmark.

Rinaldi W (1996) Understanding Ambiguity: An assessment of pragmatic meaning comprehension. Windsor: NFER-Nelson.

Rogers CR (1951) Client-centered Therapy. London: Constable.

Rondal J, Edwards S (1997) Language in Mental Retardation. London: Whurr.

Rossiter D (1997) Global outcome measures, global warning. RCSLT Bulletin 543: 8-9.

Roulstone S (1986) The speech therapist. In: Coupe J, Porter J (eds), The Education of Children with Severe Learning Difficulties. London: Croom Helm, pp. 300-311.

Royal College of Speech and Language Therapists (1996) Communicating Quality 2: Professional Standards for Speech and Language Therapists. London: RCSLT.

Royal College of Speech and Language Therapists (2001) Model of Professional Practice. London: RCSLT.

Royal College of Speech and Language Therapists (2003a) Working in Harmony. London: RCSLT.

Royal College of Speech and Language Therapists (2003b) Position Paper: Working with people with a learning difficulty. London: RCSLT.

Royal College of Speech and Language Therapists (2003c) Speech and Language Therapy Competencies, 3rd draft. London: RCSLT.

Royal College of Speech and Language Therapists (2004a) Clinical Guidelines. Bicester: Speechmark.

Royal College of Speech and Language Therapists (2004b) Newly Qualified Practititioner Competency Framework to Guide Transition to RCLST's Full Practice Register. Loondon: RCSLT.

Royal College of Speech and Language Therapists (2004c) Understanding continuing professional development. RCSLT Bull Dec.

Rustin L, Botterill W, Kelman E (1996) Assessment and Therapy for Young Dysfluent Children: Family interaction. London: Whurr.

Rustin L, Cook F, Spence R (1995) The Management of Stuttering in Adolescence: A communication skills approach. London: Whurr.

Schön D (1987) Educating the Reflective Practitioner: Toward a new design for teaching and learning in the professions. New York: Jossey-Bass.

Sears DO, Peplau A, Freedman JL, Taylor SE (1988) Social Psychology, 6th edn. Englewood Cliffs, NJ: Prentice-Hall.

Semel E, Wiig E, Secord W (1987) Clinical Evaluation of Language Fundamentals, revised edn. San Antonio: The Psychological Corporation, Harcourt Brace Jovanovich.

Sheehan JG (1975) Conflict theory and avoidance reduction therapy. In: Eisenson J (ed.), Stuttering: A second symposium. New York: Harper & Row, pp. 121-66.

Shriberg L, Lof G (1991) Reliability studies in broad and narrow phonetic transcription. Clinical Linguistics and Phonetics 5: 225-79.

Snowling M, Stackhouse J (eds) (1996) Dyslexia, Speech and Language: A practitioner's handbook. London: Whurr.

Square-Storer P (ed.) (1989) Acquired Apraxia of Speech on Adults. London: Taylor & Francis.

Stackhouse J, Wells B (1997) Children's Speech and Literacy Problems: A psycholinguistic framework. London: Whurr.

Stengelhofen J (1993) Teaching Students in Clinical Settings. London: Chapman & Hall.

Sternberg R (ed.) (1999) Handbook of Creativity. Cambridge: Cambridge University Press.

Street E (1994) Counselling for Family Problems. London: Sage.

Tuckman BW (1965) Developmental sequences in small groups. Psychological Bulletin 63: 384-99.

Turnbull J, Stewart T (1999) The Dysfluency Resource Book. Bicester: Winslow Press.

Van der Gaag A (1988) The Communication Assessment Profile for Adults with a Mental Handicap (CASP). London: Speech Profiles Ltd.

Van der Gaag A, Davies P (1992a) The professional competence of speech therapists: II Knowledge base. Clinical Rehabilitation 6: 215-24.

Van der Gaag A, Davies, P (1992b) The professional competence of speech therapists: IV Attitude and attribute base. Clinical Rehabilitation 6: 325-31.

Van Riper C (1973) The Treatment of Stuttering. Engelwood Cliffs, NJ: Prentice-Hall.

Vaughan P, Lathlean J (1999) Intermediate Care: Models in practice. London: King's Fund.

Vogel D, Carter J (1995) The Effects of Drugs on Communication Disorders. San Diego, CA: Singular Press.

Wall M, Myers F (1984) Clinical Management of Childhood Stuttering. Baltimore, MA: University Park Press.

Wertz RT, La Pointe L, Rosenbek JC (1984) Apraxia of Speech in Adults: The disorder and its management. San Diego, CA: Singular Press.

Whitaker DS (1989) Using Groups to Help People. London: Routledge.

White M, East K (1983) The Wessex Revised Portage Language Checklist. Windsor: NFER-Nelson.

Whitworth A, Perkins L, Lesser R (1997) Conversation Analysis Profile for People with Aphasia. London: Whurr.

Wilson W, Laidler P (1990) How teams can achieve 'skill blend'. Speech Therapy in Practice. December: 7-8.

Wirz S (1993) Historical considerations in assessment. In: Beech J, Harding L, Hilton-Jones D. (eds), Assessment in Speech and Language Therapy. London: Routledge, pp. 1-15.

Wirz S (1995) Perceptual Approaches to Communication Disorders. London: Whurr.

Wirz S, Beck J (1995) Assessment of voice quality: the Vocal Profiles Analysis Scheme. In: Wirz S (ed.), Perceptual Approaches to Communication Disorders. London: Whurr, pp. 39-54.

Wood S, Hardcastle B (2000) Instrumentation in the assessment and therapy of motor speech disorders: a survey of techniques and case studies with EPG. In: Papathanasiou I (ed.), Acquired Neurogenic Communication Disorders. A clinical perspective. London: Whurr, pp. 203-48.

Wootton A (1989) Speech to and from a severely retarded young Down's syndrome child. In: Beveridge M, Conti-Ramsden G, Leudar I (eds), Language and Communication in Mentally Handicapped People. London: Chapman & Hall, pp. 157–84.

World Health Organization (1979) Health for All by the Year 2000. Global strategy from 32nd World Health Assembly. Geneva: WHO.

World Health Organization (1980) International Classification of Impairments, Disabilities and Handicaps. Geneva: WHO.

World Health Organization (2001) International Classification of Functioning, Disability and Health (ICF). Geneva: WHO.

Worrall L (1999) FCTP: Functional Communication Therapy Planner. Bicester, Oxon: Winslow Press.

Wright L, Ayre A (2000) WASSP: Wright and Ayre Stuttering Self-Rating Profile. Bicester, Oxon: Winslow Press.

Index

Lightning Source UK Ltd.
Milton Keynes UK
05 September 2010

159422UK00002B/7/P